Praise for *Recover!*

"*Recover!* provides an astonishing array of resources, neatly organized into accessible and sensible tasks, and a final chapter for coping with unexpected problems. In this book you will find guidance on everything you need to address in recovery. Stanton Peele doesn't tell you what to do, but shows you the tasks that need to be accomplished and gives you options for moving forward."

—Tom Horvath, PhD, ABPP; President, Smart Recovery® and Practical Recovery

"Stanton Peele has long been at the forefront of the battle to understand addictions and eliminate the twin myths that addicts are powerless over their addictions and that they have a lifelong 'brain disease.' In *Recover!* he has taken another crucial step toward freeing us from these prejudicial, disempowering misconceptions while truly helping people suffering with addiction."

—Lance Dodes, MD, Assistant Clinical Professor of Psychiatry, Harvard Medical School (retired); author of *Breaking Addiction* and *The Heart of Addiction*

"At a time when addiction is being trumpeted as a 'brain disease,' Peele slashes through the hypermedicalized rhetoric to get to the human core of addiction and recovery. This acutely insightful and compassionate book is required reading for anyone struggling with an overwhelming habit."

—Sally Satel, MD, coauthor of *Brainwashed: The Seductive Appeal of Mindless Neuroscience*; lecturer, Yale University School of Medicine

"I have known Stanton Peele over the decades as one of the great addiction theorists. In *Recover!* I rediscover him as an absolutely down-to-earth personal counselor who makes me understand mindfulness in an entirely different way. Great book!"

—Bruce Alexander, Rat Park experimenter; author, *The Globalization of Addiction*

"Stanton Peele's insistence that addiction is not a disease, but a symptom of dysfunctional societies, families, and/or psyches is compelling, compassionate, and almost certainly correct. In *Recover!*, his most impressive work to date, he lays out a program—both utterly simple and profound—that will quite literally save lives by addressing the root causes of addiction rather than pathologizing its many manifestations."

—Christopher Ryan, Ph.D. & Cacilda Jethá, M.D., authors of the *New York Times* bestseller *Sex at Dawn*

"12-step treatment worsened my addiction to the point that I nearly died of withdrawal. Stanton Peele's books saved my life by showing me that I was not powerless and did not need to be rescued by a 'Higher Power.' For a step-by-step guide on how to overcome addiction I most highly recommend Dr. Peele's new book *Recover!*"

—Kenneth Anderson, MA, Founder and CEO of HAMS Harm Reduction for Alcohol

"In *Recover!*, Stanton Peele and Ilse Thompson offer a blueprint to help addicts cope with their triggers, from loneliness and feeling unworthy, anxious, and overwhelmed. *Recover!* focuses on what's *right* in the addict's life, and adding to it. It's a hopeful, tangible set of tools designed to give power back to the addict—not give it up."

—Gabrielle Glaser, author of the *New York Times* bestseller *Her Best-Kept Secret: Why Women Drink—And How They Can Regain Control*

"'I am a recovering addict' was the way someone introduced himself to me on my first visit to the USA. He explained he had been in recovery for the past 25 years. The irrationality, helplessness and disempowerment inherent in this statement shocked me. This is what the disease model of addiction does to people. I am in agreement with Stanton Peele that people are not powerless or helpless in the face of dependence on drugs, and the evidence supports this view. This book dispels that, and other myths about drugs. Stanton has come up with another must-read book."

—Professor Pat O'Hare, co-founder and former director of Harm Reduction International

"Stanton Peele's writing has been a Copernican paradigm shift in the field of recovery. With his *Diseasing of America*, Peele emerged as a savvy provocateur with the guts to take on the recovery establishment. With *Recover!* Peele shares his clinical wisdom and compassion with those who are on the path of change and self-acceptance. *Recover!* is a recovery program of practical perfection without the typical recovery perfectionism."

—Pavel Somov, Ph.D., author of *Lotus Effect* and *Eating the Moment: 141 Mindful Practices to Overcome Overeating One Meal at a Time*

"*Recover!* is a powerful new tool for helping people with addictions heal and grow. Dr. Stanton Peele is a trailblazer who has led each new progressive wave in the addictive behaviors field since the 1970s. Today, Dr. Peele is a leading voice for a new shift in the field, one that refutes the myth that addicted people are victims of a permanent disease that they can arrest only by accepting their powerlessness and lifelong abstinence. *Recover!* is a how-to guide to recovery through cultivating mindful awareness and self-compassion. Inspiring, hopeful, and a good read as well."

—Andrew Tatarsky, PhD, author, *Harm Reduction Psychotherapy: A New Treatment for Drug and Alcohol Problems*; Director, Center for Optimal Living, NYC

"In the midst of the turbulence about defining and dealing with addiction, Stanton Peele has consistently articulated one of the few sane voices. Increasingly, research has proved that he is right. *Recover!* continues and extends his presence at the forefront of advice and help based on common sense and efficacy for those struggling with addiction."

—Liese Recke, Manager of Clinical Treatment, Oslo Norway, and former addict

"Probably the world's most notable figure in addiction studies, Stanton Peele has written another great book. *Recover!* really is a self-help book. Unlike most of what you read, it teaches you to help yourself, rather than telling you to rely on a treatment system because helping oneself is impossible. Stanton's work assisted my recovery many years ago, and he can help you now."

—Peter Ferentzy, Ph.D., author of *Dealing with an Addict: What You Need to Know if Someone You Care for Has a Drug or Alcohol Problem*

"Stanton Peele knows more about addiction than anyone in the world. Every one of his books is a masterpiece. So is this one. The materials in this book are factual, inspiring and helpful for anyone making for change on their own. If you need additional help, take this book to a good therapist. Ask them to help you apply Peele's materials. You will be very happy with the results!"

—Robert M. Muscala, R.N., Addiction/Chemical Health Specialist, Minnesota

Praise for Stanton Peele

"There were two books that really had a significant impact on me on the issue of drugs: One was Andrew Weil's book, *The Natural Mind*. The second book that really made an impact on me was Stanton Peele's *The Meaning of Addiction*."

—Ethan Nadelmann, Ph.D., Founder and Director of Drug Policy Alliance, the primary drug policy reform organization in the U.S.

"Peele offers mindful alternatives to those suffering from addictions and to professionals seeking to help them."

—Ellen Langer, Department of Psychology, Harvard University; author of *Mindfulness* and *Counterclockwise: Mindful Health and the Power of Possibility*

"I read *Love and Addiction* as soon as it was published. It was probably the first book I ever read which analyzed addiction in a way that made sense to me and echoed what I knew from my work. Years later, I undertook a study looking at recovered addicts who had been sexually abused as children. I pulled *Love and Addiction* off the shelf. It still reads absolutely true as an understanding of addictive behavior all these years later."

—Rowdy Yates, Ph.D., Department of Addiction Studies, University of Stirling

"*The Truth About Addiction and Recovery* is an unusually well-researched and persuasively presented book on some of the main myths about addiction and recovery. Required reading for addicts, their associates, and those who try to treat them."

—Albert Ellis, Ph.D., founder of Rational-Emotive Therapy; ranked in a survey of psychologists as the second most influential psychotherapist in history

"Stanton Peele is the only author who has effectively challenged the consistent failure of the mental health establishment, the huge AA and Synanon-type 'religions,' the drug enforcement bureaucracy, and the medical profession."

—Nicholas Cummings, Ph.D., Past President, American Psychological Association; Chief of Mental Health, Kaiser Permanente Health Maintenance Organization

"*Diseasing of America* is a provocative review of the uses and abuses of the disease model in the past three decades. This important book has significantly added to my education and clinical understanding of addiction in my professional practice."

—Richard R. Irons, M.D., FASAM, The Menninger Clinic

"Peele makes it clear that the disease model of addiction is an emperor without clothes. By placing addictive behaviors in the context of other problems of living, he emphasizes personal responsibility for one's habits. The book empowers the reader to view addiction in a new optimistic light."

—G. Alan Marlatt, founder of Addictive Behaviors Research Center, University of Washington; co-editor of *Relapse Prevention*

"Dr. Peele's work has influenced my professional work and changed my personal life for the better."

—Anne M. Fletcher, M.S., R.D., L.D., author of *Thin for Life*, *Sober for Good*, and *Inside Rehab: The Surprising Truth About Addiction Treatment—and How to Get Help That Works*

"We have more than enough diseases without inventing new ones to relieve us of moral responsibility to deal with the complexity of the human condition. *Diseasing of America* is an important book that should be read by all concerned about addiction. An added bonus—Dr. Peele writes exceptionally well."

—Neil A. Kurtzman, M.D., Chairman, Department of Internal Medicine, Texas Tech University Health Sciences Center

Recover!

Also by Stanton Peele

7 Tools to Beat Addiction

Love and Addiction
(with Archie Brodsky)

How Much Is Too Much

Addiction-Proof Your Child

The Science of Experience

The Meaning of Addiction

Visions of Addiction
(edited volume)

Diseasing of America

The Truth About Addiction and Recovery
(with Archie Brodsky and Mary Arnold)

Alcohol and Pleasure
(edited volume, with Marcus Grant)

Resisting 12-Step Coercion
(with Charles Bufe and Archie Brodsky)

An Empowering Program to Help You Stop Thinking Like an Addict and **Reclaim Your Life**

STANTON PEELE, Ph.D.

with ILSE THOMPSON

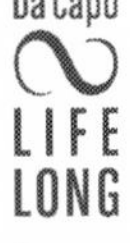

A Member of the Perseus Books Group

 For information, address Da Capo Press, 44 Farnsworth Street, 3rd Floor, Boston, MA 02210

Designed by Cynthia Young

Cataloging-in-Publication data for this book is available from the Library of Congress.

First Da Capo Press edition 2014
First Da Capo Press paperback edition 2015

ISBN: 978-0-7382-1675-1 (hardcover)
ISBN: 978-0-7382-1812-0 (paperback)
ISBN: 978-0-7382-1676-8 (e-book)

Published by Da Capo Press
A Member of the Perseus Books Group
www.dacapopress.com

Note: The information in this book is true and complete to the best of our knowledge. This book is intended only as an informative guide for those wishing to know more about health issues. In no way is this book intended to replace, countermand, or conflict with the advice given to you by your own physician or therapist, if you currently have or plan to consult with one. The ultimate decisions concerning care should be made between you and your doctor and therapist. We strongly recommend you discuss any actions you plan to take as a result of reading this book with either your physician or therapist, if you currently have or plan to consult with one, and keep any health care professional with whom you consult informed about the actions you take and your ongoing health and mental health status. Information in this book is general and is offered with no guarantees on the part of the authors or Da Capo Press. The authors and publisher disclaim all liability in connection with the use of this book.

To the memory of Alan Marlatt
Always at the forefront

Contents

Acknowledgments

I thank primarily two people for their help in writing this book. Ilse Thompson, whose role is acknowledged on the title page, did significant original thinking and writing, especially concerning the linkage between the downsides of current American practice regarding addiction and an alternative way of conceiving of humanity in relation to addiction and righting people's relationship to the universe. Ilse is a treasured colleague and friend—moreover, one whose efforts on our joint behalf never flagged. Her contributions to this book, from start to finish, are invaluable, incalculable, and irreplaceable—*Recover!* would not exist without her.

And, as always, Archie Brodsky played an essential role in conceiving and executing *Recover!* Since we worked together to write *Love and Addiction*, published in 1975, Archie has helped with every major project I have embarked on—and not only writing projects. No idea or word that appears in the book has escaped his attention. Archie's wife, Vicki Rowland, played a vital part in our working sessions, contributing insights and technical resourcefulness along with unflagging hospitality during my visits to Archie's and her home.

Along the way, a remarkable number of people have made inputs, read sections of the book, corrected my misunderstandings, and tried to help in any way they could. This list includes Chris Ryan, Alan Cudmore, Ruth Gasparik, Sylvia Carlson, Mylissa Emrick, Kenneth Anderson, Adi Jaffe, Nona Jordan, Maia Szalavitz, Alta Ann Parkins Morris, and others I may have missed.

My editor Renée Sedliar and agent Andrew Stuart have been steadfastly supportive in the always-challenging enterprise of creating a book. Their calm confidence, good spirits, and good judgment have buoyed Ilse and me whenever necessary—which has been more than once. In our editorial exchanges Renée has managed to be both consistently encouraging and helpfully critical. Also in our corner have been Merloyd Lawrence, Renée's colleague and a longtime supporter of Archie's and mine, and Hara Marano, *Psychology Today* editor-at-large and longtime friend and colleague. Hara—who both assisted me in publishing my work in *Psychology Today* magazine over five separate decades and with Lybi Ma enabled me to garner several million readers of my posts at *Psychology Today* Blogs*—introduced me to her and now my agent, Andrew, and thus started the process of publishing *Recover!*.

At any age, but especially now, it is both important and extremely gratifying to have people—more than those named—who wish me well and who want to see my ideas reach and help more people. Thank you.

Stanton Peele
November 2013

* I am likewise exceedingly grateful to the *Huffington Post* for giving me an equally visible and positive platform to present my ideas about addiction and much else.

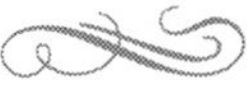

Introduction

What *Recover!* is about, and how to use this book

This book is written to clarify what addiction is, and how you or a loved one can overcome it. You are coming to this book for one of three reasons: to deal effectively with your own addiction, to help someone you care about who struggles with addictive problems, or out of interest in and curiosity about the subject.

There are two competing views of addiction out there. The one you are used to hearing is that addiction is a disease, meaning that it is a biological force over which you have no control. This is what we have been told for decades. This view is wrong.

The other view, which is the basis for The PERFECT Program outlined in this book, is that addiction is a natural but destructive expression of a person's outlook in reaction to his or her life circumstances. I will show that this view is scientifically valid, true to life, and much more helpful than the disease view. People get themselves into addictions for understandable reasons, and people can get themselves out by being mindful of who they are and who they can and want to be.

The title *Recover!* is in the form of an imperative because you need to know that you will recover if you follow the typical path addicts experience. Science tells us this. You need to know this truth to clear away the underbrush impeding your recovery and to maximize your chance to recover—not to mention expedite the process—which requires that you galvanize your own resources. This book is the manual for how to accomplish your own recovery.

This way of looking at addiction makes possible an entirely different approach to overcoming addictions, one that is both more hopeful and more practical. It plays to your strengths, not weaknesses. But before I present this empowering approach to addiction, you need to discard some myths, old and new, about addiction.

Contrary to the medical-sounding idea of addiction as a "disease," the 12-step catechism of Alcoholics Anonymous originated in America's deeply held fears of alcohol (and later, other drugs) and is steeped in religious ideas and irrationality. Why, then, have you been hearing so much lately about brain science proving that addiction is a disease? Neurobiological studies of dopamine and the limbic system do little to inform us of the ways and means to overcome an addiction, and they most assuredly do not justify a 12-step approach that appeals to God to cure your disease.

Moreover, how does it help you to believe that your brain can be "hijacked" by addiction—a highly publicized, supposedly scientific idea? If that were so, then people wouldn't be able to wait until break time to go outside to smoke, or they wouldn't only resort to their drug addiction in the company of certain people and in certain places. In fact, addicts exercise control over their addictions all the time, and most addicts outgrow their addictions. It is also true that everyone experiences an addiction in their own way, and everyone must—and can—find their own way out of addiction.

By reinforcing the myth that addiction is uncontrollable and permanent, neuroscientific models make it *harder* to overcome the problem, just as the 12-step disease model has all along. Telling yourself that you are "powerless" over addiction is self-defeating; it limits your capacity to change and grow. Isn't it better to start from the belief that you—or your spouse, or your child—can fully and finally break out of addictive habits by redirecting your life? It may not be quick and easy to accomplish, but it happens all the time. In this book I will show you how it happens and what it takes to do it.

Mindfulness is a key component of The PERFECT Program. It is both a Buddhist and a modern psychological concept. Combining the two, mindfulness means being in the moment by being aware of your circumstances—your surroundings, yourself, the here and now—all of which determine how you feel and act. It strengthens your ability to bring into your consciousness the key elements of your addiction—your motivation, your situation, your needs, and your ability to make alternative choices. Mindfulness gives you the space, the ability, and the self-confidence to outgrow your addiction. You can improve this ability, as you can any mental or physical capacity, by learning about and practicing it—including using the meditations provided throughout this book.

One claim often made for the disease theory of addiction, now dressed up in neuroscience, is that explaining the cause of your addiction as being outside your control frees you of guilt. Yes, but at the cost of telling you that you are a slave to your addiction. The PERFECT Program invites self-acceptance, or the belief in your underlying value—troubled as you may be—as a human being. For it is only by combining mindfulness—genuine awareness—with faith in yourself that you can finally empower yourself to grow beyond addiction. This process entails self-acceptance, another modern version of a Buddhist concept, this one called loving kindness.

The PERFECT Program allows you to achieve a better life not by *escaping* anything, but rather by *embracing* who you are, who you wish to be, and who you can be. Regarding yourself as "perfect"—yet another Buddhist idea—again corresponds with the best contemporary psychological thinking. Embracing your perfection (which is not the same as smug self-satisfaction and denial) encourages your faith in your ability to change and accelerates the change process.

Here is a concrete example of the difference between AA's disease theory and The PERFECT Program. AA's first step commands you to accept that you are powerless: "We admitted we were powerless over our addiction—that our lives had become unmanageable." Step One, then, is the justification for the cadres of counselors who come down like a ton of bricks on addicts in treatment programs, telling them that they can't manage their lives. In other words, if you are addicted, that is all you are, and your life has become worthless, and only the "helpers" can make you whole.

The PERFECT Program rejects this kind of thinking, expressed in the self-labeling mantra, "I am an addict." It starts instead from two assumptions: every human being is already worthwhile, and you will succeed best when you feel best about yourself, your potential, and your core value. You still need to take responsibility for your actions and practice the discipline required to put your life on track. But you are not your addiction;

you are a valuable human being whose qualities endure and exceed your addiction.

These fundamental differences translate into different helping techniques. Instead of focusing solely on the object of addiction and its all-conquering force, as AA and neuroscience do, The PERFECT Program directs you to contemplate your addiction from a broader perspective that takes in your life history, environmental influences, and personal relationships, as well as your feelings, beliefs, and outlooks.

Addicts regularly respond to challenging situations by panicking—after all, they have "admitted" that they are incapable of managing their lives. The most natural immediate reaction when you are so overwhelmed is to resume your addiction—or else seek protective refuge in the group (the 12-step solution). The PERFECT Program instead helps you manage stress and anxiety without resorting to your addiction. The PERFECT Program believes you *can* help yourself—indeed, it is *based* on the assumption that you are the crucial, the only, agent of your own change.

How to Use This Book

Recover! is divided into two parts. The first part of the book is an orientation for people with addiction problems and also for people who want to get inside the mind of an addict. Part I prepares you for The PERFECT Program. It provides first the story of a methamphetamine addict, Rose, so that you can understand the personal experience of addiction and recovery through the eyes of one woman. It then presents a history and scientific understanding of addiction, so that you will know what it is that you are confronting and how often—and how—people overcome it. This section is less prescriptive, and sometimes less experiential and more expository, than the second part of the book, which prepares you to embark on PERFECT and then presents The PERFECT Program itself. If you are coming to this book for help with an addiction, since you have your own addiction narrative, you may feel that Rose's story in Chapter 1 isn't relevant, or that the analysis in Chapter 2 isn't for you. You may be tempted to jump ahead to Part II and directly into PERFECT. But, be assured, there is value for you in these early chapters as preparation for launching The PERFECT Program—not least in getting out from under the dead weight of misguided and counterproductive ideas.

Please also note that, while the nature of a book requires that it progress in some logical order, you will have a path out of addiction that is unique to you. You may have to linger longer in some phases of PERFECT; some parts may be more difficult for you to practice than others. Fine, this isn't a race. At the same time, Chapter 10, "Triage," is your go-to chapter for crisis moments. If you find yourself at a loss or in urgent need, jump right into that chapter as your immediate reference and guide to your options.

Taken as a whole, The PERFECT Program demystifies addiction. It offers a practical application of the best research, neutralizes the mythological power of inert substances and self-destructive behaviors, and gives you the knowledge and power to express intentionally the freedom you already sense inside you. It is a self-directed process of fortifying your life from the ground up and making addiction obsolete. It's an accessible, layered program, based on what we know to be true about addiction and what has been proven to overcome it.

The tools we offer you to achieve freedom are a synthesis of the best practices for changing how you respond to addictive urges, developing the skills to live fully and prevent relapse, and replacing paralyzing assumptions with positive options. Through PERFECT, you will learn new habits of mind and heart that reclaim your genuine self, expand and strengthen your life skills, and embrace a life of engagement, meaning, and purpose.

The origins of addiction are as complex and unique as the people who find themselves in its grip. But rather than homing in on what may have gone wrong in your life, The PERFECT Program teaches you how to build the foundation of your recovery on *what's already right.* You have a healthy inner core that instinctively rejects self-destructive behavior. You know this; you hear it cry out time and again. It may even have caused you to try to quit—and to quit for a time. People are often discouraged when they fail to stay off an addiction, and such setbacks are often used to prove they have a disease they will never overcome. In fact, however, having quit previously for a time is a *positive predictor that you will recover.*[1] Efforts at quitting show the most important thing about you in relation to your addiction—that you *want* to quit.

The PERFECT Program is presented in Part II in seven chapters, preceded by the preparations and materials you will need. Each chapter lays out a distinct part of the program that corresponds to a letter in the acronym "PERFECT." These chapters incorporate three phases of change you will undergo: foundational (deep inner work), structural (creating a framework of life skills and values), and operational (living with balance and intention). Each chapter lays out clear goals for you to pursue, journal exercises, guided meditations, progress tracking, and other powerful tools you can use in your daily life. So, hear this: you are *not* a passive spectator to your brain's functioning or an unfortunate victim of it. You are the primary generator of how your brain functions—of how you function—both in the here and now, and certainly over the long run.

PAUSE

Mindfulness—Learning to listen to yourself

EMBRACE

Self-acceptance and forgiveness—Learning to love yourself

REDISCOVER

Integrity—Finding and following your true self

FORTIFY

Coping—Learning the skills for life management

EMBARK

Equilibrium—Proceeding on an even keel

CELEBRATE

Joy—Honoring your accomplishments and milestones

TRIAGE

Realignment—Resources and actions for regaining lost footing

To show how PERFECT works and to get you started, "P" stands for "Pause"—a mark of mindfulness. This pause allows you to establish your calm inner essence. It also gives you space to consider your options—including rediscovering and mobilizing your core resources. PERFECT focuses you on those things you know how to do, and to do well, so that you can generalize the competence and confidence you feel in these areas and build on hard-won feelings of self-worth and capability. Let's say you are an excellent car mechanic or athlete—you can borrow the skills and self-command you bring to bear on these activities into areas where you feel insecure and perform poorly, so that you become less likely to turn to an addiction.

After and along with pausing to consider and apply your mind to a problem, you "Embrace" (the "E" in PERFECT). Whom and what do you embrace? Yourself and all that you stand for and can do, now and in the future. *Embrace* embodies the critical psychological idea of self-acceptance, which—along with mindfulness—is the essential foundation for living free of addiction. As with other key tools in *Recover!* this is a contemporary psychological idea that corresponds closely to a Buddhist-inspired concept—that of "loving kindness." In addition to compassion for yourself, loving kindness conveys compassion for others—which leads in turn to forgiveness.

The absence of self-acceptance—in fact, the indoctrination in its opposite—is the worst thing about the 12 steps. As practiced in addiction treatment throughout the United States, the steps hammer home that you are not worthy of your own and others' love. Self-acceptance, which takes you in the opposite direction from this self-denigration, is at the heart of The PERFECT Program.

Used as a guide for applying mindfulness and self-acceptance, *Recover!* is your manual for asserting your power to overcome your addiction. In the following chapters, you can prepare for, then proceed mindfully through, The PERFECT Program and into your addiction-free life.

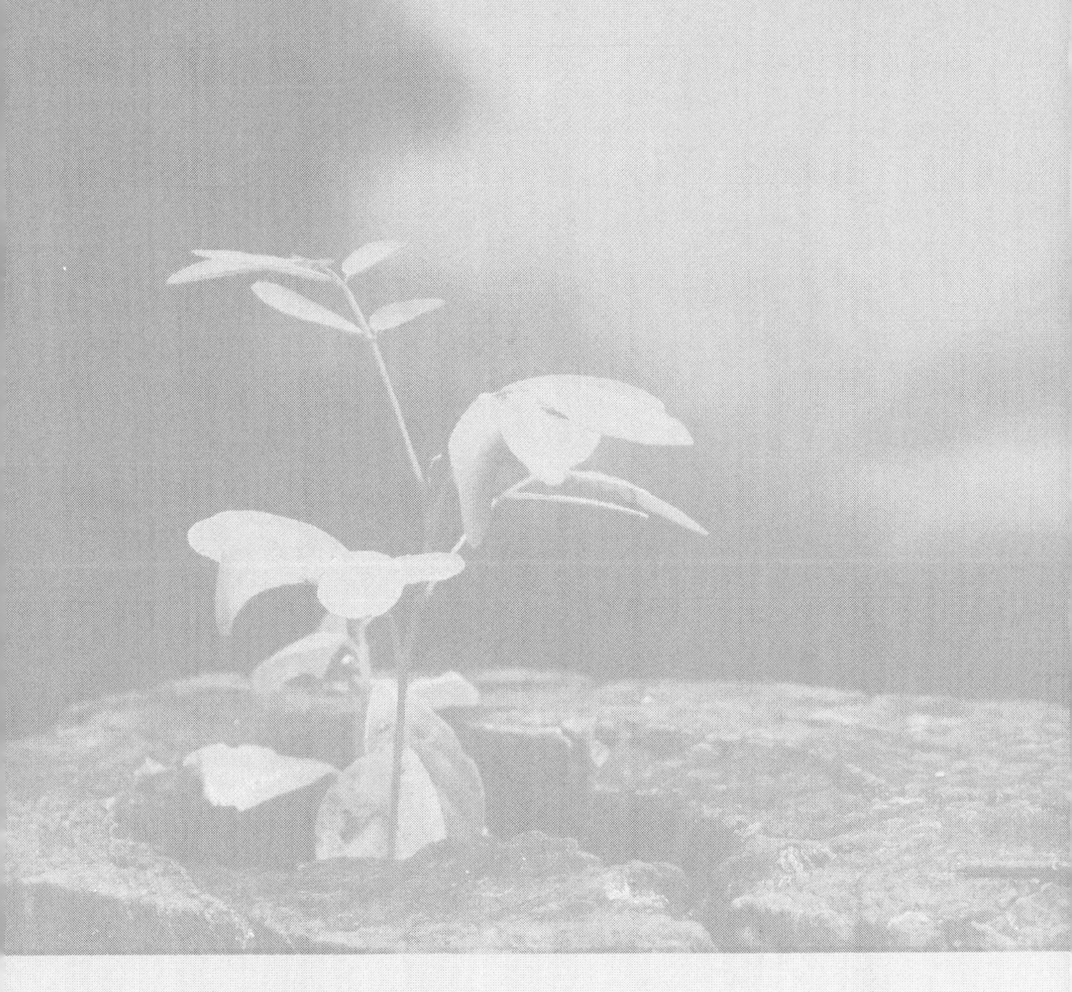

PART I
THE MEANING OF ADDICTION AND RECOVERY

CHAPTER 1

The Story of Rose—An Addict

How one becomes an addict, then recovers

CHAPTER GOALS

- To describe what an addict's life looks like
- To understand what caused her addiction—what does she *get* from it?
- To learn whether she is doomed if she doesn't get with the 12 steps
- To trace how she recovered through The PERFECT Program approach
- To learn how to apply these insights to your own addiction

Purpose: In order to combat addiction, for yourself, for a loved one, or in society as a whole, you need to see into the heart of addiction. This chapter will put you inside the mind of an addict, Rose, so that you can understand and appreciate her life and her thinking, and then will show you how she emerged from addiction through the course of her life. In this way, Rose is showing the way for you—for all of us. Although Rose was addicted to meth—what some consider to be a "real" addiction (a distinction with no meaning)—her story illustrates *all* addiction and recovery. Perhaps you'll find similarities between Rose's story and yours, regardless of the particular substance or activity to which you may be addicted. What's important for you is how Rose used The PERFECT Program to overcome addiction.

To illustrate both how and why people become addicted, and how people recover according to the principles and practices of The PERFECT Program, consider Rose, who became an injecting meth addict. Rose was sidetracked from a promising academic career by an unexpected pregnancy. Weighed down by demands of part-time college attendance, single parenthood, and work, she turned to meth (also known as "speed," "crank," and "ice") for a "pick-me-up" to enable her to carry through her responsibilities, and especially her obligations to her daughter, to whom she was committed above all else.

Struggling to support herself and her daughter, Rose felt constantly exhausted and on the verge of a breakdown. Her grades in college were marginal, not because she wasn't a good student but because she couldn't find enough time and energy to study. Meth seemed to offer redemption. After first taking meth, Rose felt invincible. She immediately cleaned her entire apartment. Stunned by how much she had accomplished—it was still only 3 a.m.—she brought out her textbooks and started working on her school assignments. At 6 a.m., done! By the time the sun came up Rose had formulated a new strategy for achieving the goals she had set for herself and her daughter. She saw the drug as giving a boost to her productivity and contentment so that she could carry the weight of her combined obligations. When the school year was over she would quit the drug, Rose figured.

And meth served her purposes for a time. But given the stress in Rose's life, this balance didn't hold. Gradually, she stopped getting high to accomplish things. Instead, getting high became a goal in itself. Now she pushed her responsibilities aside to make time for her drug use. As the drug took center stage in her life, Rose fell farther behind, and she started to lose the things that were important to her. She abandoned her schooling, the reason she thought she began taking meth in the first place. Then she cut back her working hours. Although her co-workers could see that something was amiss, Rose still managed to be responsible—only now for limited periods of time, after which she turned to her drug of choice. It was all she could do to hold on.

When meth started to become her first priority, fearing her own behavior, Rose sent her daughter to live with her parents for a *temporary* period (as she imagined it). It wasn't so much that she neglected her child as that she was overcome with worry that her daughter would notice something was wrong with her mother. This created in Rose a constant sense of shame whenever she looked at her child. But, of course, with her daughter gone, Rose could now use the drug without constraints. She associated exclusively with people who shared her use of meth. Her inhibitions lowered and her adrenaline elevated, she found it easy to make seemingly profound connections with other users, especially men. After spending all day and night talking nonstop, the interactions often turned sexual. But the deep connections she thought she was making invariably turned out to be one-night stands.

Now she was taking the drug to feel alive and well, perhaps to hook up and feel—if not loved—at least desirable, and to forget her actual state of affairs. Rose no longer had any other way to make life seem okay to her. She deteriorated physically: her skin was an eerie shade of gray, marred by eruptions. She lost twenty pounds. *Who could find me attractive now*, she thought, with what insight remained to her.

Although she experienced panic attacks, Rose viewed sleep as an enemy to be avoided at all costs. She ignored the normal sequence of nights following days, since her energy came from a drug that disregarded the usual time schedules. Her user friends were awake and busy 24/7. Days went by at hyper-speed, and she couldn't recall how many nights she had been awake. When her body and mind could not be pushed farther, Rose crashed. She and her friends often passed out in the middle of a sentence, dropped what they were holding, and fell asleep. Upon awakening, Rose repeated the whole process—using, staying up for days on end, then falling into a stupor.

By now, Rose no longer gained the level of energy and feelings of escape that had formed the experience to which she had become addicted—she had seemingly become immune to the drug's familiar effects. Instead of feeling nonstop motivation, staying up all night getting things done, Rose now needed the drug just to conduct daily activities—she could no longer wake up and start a day without speed. At this point, Rose began injecting—rather than snorting—the drug. Rose's problem had morphed into self-induced narcolepsy, for which the only antidote was methamphetamine. She felt like she had become the victim of a kind of bait and switch—that the drug and its effects had defrauded her!

Each time Rose injected, she was filled with revulsion and guilt. Yet she carried on. She wished for a do-over; she promised herself that she was going to stop as soon as she finished the drugs she had on hand. Or next week. Or as soon as she found a better job. Rose missed her child more than anything. When it was time to go home for a visit, Rose obsessively primped her hair and makeup so that, she forlornly hoped, nothing would seem amiss to her daughter or her parents. Of course, they knew something was wrong, and Rose knew that they knew.

Then she returned, guilt in hand, to her apartment and her drug. Despite her painful moments of awareness, the drag of addiction always managed to pull her back under. The regret and guilt of using in and of itself, especially after she began injecting, became her major motivation to use, since she was overwhelmed with a sense of dread when the effects of the drug wore off. Thinking of what she had given up to her addiction—primarily her daughter—triggered a pain for which she had only one remedy: meth. Rose could not see any way out of this mess. At least by using, she got relief for a time from her overwhelming emotional pain and guilt. She *needed* to return to her drugged state. It was, in a paradoxical way, her comfort zone.

Because Rose failed to act against her addiction, she thought this proved her drug use was an illness. After all, everyone knew that drug addicts are powerless and out of control. That message was reinforced when Rose for a time attended 12-step meetings—the only way she knew of to begin to address her problem. Rose came to believe she was not a normal person and could never be one, just a recovering person. But whenever she contemplated recovery, she rejected it. It was overwhelming and demoralizing: detox, rehab, meetings, steps—*forever*. Although what she was doing was no life for her, neither were the 12 steps. Besides, she knew so many people who cycled through recovery programs that she and her friends joked: "Joe's in the spin-dry. He'll be back any day now."

With her addiction now so disabling, Rose decided not to attend her daughter's fifth birthday party. She couldn't stomach the masquerade and, mostly, didn't want to face the emotional pain of being a bystander at the event. Then, for weeks afterwards, she regretted missing this milestone in her child's life. This must mean she had hit "rock bottom" (a meaningless term to which we will return). Some time after that, she was revolted by what she saw in the mirror. *I'm far gone*, she thought. Rose was hooked, without a doubt, especially since she had progressed from snorting the drug to shooting it intravenously in order to get more bang for her ever-diminishing buck. Her self-disgust and fear were now without bounds.

Missing her daughter's birthday party had a special impact for Rose, and her thoughts constantly returned to it. It made clear to Rose, as nothing else could, that the costs of her drug use outweighed any benefits that remained from it—even as this would have been obvious all along to anyone with an outside perspective. This experience, for Rose, finally made it intolerable for her to consider getting high. Rose didn't take the drug one day when she usually would have. She pulled out her daughter's pictures and mementos to give her a touchstone to cement her commitment to quitting. As one day without meth stretched to two, Rose was as amazed as anyone could have been that she didn't use. She had almost unintentionally detoxed, something she had always feared she could not do.

At first, Rose simply slept hard, then woke up angry. Then she slept more. She was ravenous, but didn't have the energy or the stomach to eat. Nonetheless, every hour she passed without getting high was as precious as gold in the bank, and each deposit made the idea of cashing out harder to conceive. When Rose felt that the worst of it had passed, she called her mother. As terrified as her mother had become through Rose's whole ordeal (the dimensions of which she could only surmise), she began crying as Rose explained what had been going on and asked her for help. Her mom came over with a homemade meal. Together they came up with a plan for Rose to reestablish her life, placing what was important at its center.

It might seem strange that Rose could form such ideas so quickly. But, really, they had been floating through her mind all along. All addicts have some kind of alternative, non-addicted identity waiting to surface. For Rose, this identity was always with her. Before she ever became hooked on meth, Rose felt that she was failing at what was most important to her: creating a comfortable, secure life for her daughter. Everything she did by working and going to school had been in the interest of achieving that dream, which somehow always exceeded her capacity.

With what she was struggling to achieve firmly reestablished in her mind, Rose moved back into her parents' house, rejoining her daughter's daily life. Rose returned to school and found a part-time job at a dentist's office (which was good, because she required considerable dental work).[1] Although she had given up quite a bit of freedom, Rose now shared childcare responsibilities while living with her parents, and that support took enough of the burden off her that she could pursue her studies while sustaining her recovery from addiction. This arrangement contrasted with the level of responsibility Rose had previously thought she could assume as a single parent and student, but that had created an imbalanced life (too much output, not enough reward), which, in turn, had primed her for addiction.

All of this was by no means an easy journey for Rose. In addition to the painful way she had arrived at her current resolution, Rose still struggled with depression when she thought of what she had done and how far behind she had fallen. Her thoughts would sometimes sneak back to the drug, romanticizing her former life. But she quickly regained perspective and realized how really dreadful her life actually had become.

Most important was that Rose was able to see the positive results of her changed life and to savor being clean. She was living in harmony with the goals that had been eluding her even before she became addicted. Rose was able to fit both play and quality time with her child into her schedule, as well as spending time with her family. Given where she was coming from, the situation seemed like a dream come true. Beyond this, Rose made space to run and do yoga. Her new circumstances honored the vision she had been working so hard for before her addiction. Now every facet of her life reflected her heart and brought her sense of purpose into sharper focus. She was using her values as a guide to create a place in the world for herself that she had dreamed of.

After quitting meth, Rose began attending an Alcoholics Anonymous group in a church near her parents' home. But if she had hated the 12-step meetings she attended before, they seemed worse to her now. How could it be good for her to feel that she was powerless over her addiction after she had just quit meth? That made no sense. But these people were the experts, she thought, and their ideas worried her. Rose also entered a community program run by recovering addicts. There she always got the impression that she was a broken, horrible, incapable person whose core elements had to be ripped down and rebuilt according to a standard only the long-recovering addicts understood. She hated that feeling. Rose left the program and AA.

Instead, Rose started attending a group for single mothers. She found that many of these women shared the same feelings of helplessness and loss of control that she had succumbed to, even if they hadn't become crank addicts. Feeling deeply ashamed, she finally brought up her former addiction to the group. It was a surprise to Rose when the other women told her that quitting meth the way she had was remarkable, and something she should be deeply proud of. Nor did they quibble with her having done so without 12-step support.

Rose also started seeing a psychologist. This woman didn't follow the 12 steps. Instead, she worked on Rose's self-esteem, which was essential to rebuilding her mothering and other skills. Rose used her therapy in support of turning her life around, of changing its entire trajectory. She progressed in school and later got a job that made use of her skills as she moved into a good career. In her late thirties now, she fell in love with a man and married him. Of course, despite the crushing addiction she experienced, there is quite a bit of life left for Rose, as there is for you.

* * *

We see in Rose's case the basis of an addict's experience—the stressful, overwhelming situation leading to drug use, then dependence on the drug; her sense of inadequacy and guilt; needing the rewards provided by the drug even *after* these became a substitute for true satisfaction and instead caused further degradation. Yet somehow the addiction *protected* Rose from recognizing how far she had fallen and how degraded her life had become. More important, we see through Rose's case the essential elements that led to her recovery, a recovery not dependent on an addiction-focused support group or belief system, other than a belief in herself and in the life she could create for herself and her daughter. For Rose, this meant learning to live her life in the moment, being aware of what the world had to offer her, while becoming aware of how her addiction deprived her of these pleasures and opportunities. The fundamental elements of recovery for Rose were her values, derailed for a time, then recaptured; the support and help she got from her parents, her group for single mothers, and her therapist; and her purpose in life—her love for her daughter and a desire to further her and her daughter's life together.

You can use this method, too, by incorporating the values, purpose, motivation, support, skills, and—underlying these—the mindfulness and self-acceptance that comprise The PERFECT Program. Your story may differ substantially from Rose's. After all, you may not be addicted to a powerful illicit street drug, and you may not be able to move back with your parents as Rose could. But, in other ways, the path you travel may be quite similar to hers. *Recover!* will enable you, like Rose, to reach into yourself and look around you in a mindful way to find all the elements of a satisfying, constructive, connected life that are essential for true recovery. *Recover!* will also help you do another thing Rose did: to replace self-doubt and searing self-criticism with self-acceptance and self-love.

CHAPTER 2

Explaining Addiction and Recovery

How Americans learn to think like addicts; how to stop

CHAPTER GOALS

- To understand what addiction is
- To learn how the disease model originated and perpetuates itself
- To grasp the downsides of thinking that your addiction is a disease
- To examine the implications—pro and con—of the new brain science
- To learn that people usually recover—why and how they do so
- To recognize your resources for recovery and launch PERFECT

Purpose: This chapter discusses how we have come to think about addiction the way we do—and how this isn't dictated by science, but by American tradition and cultural ways of thinking. It will take you through the history of the development of the disease concept of addiction, how this idea has been sold as "science" but (1) isn't science and (2) isn't helpful. You will learn that nothing is more natural than recovery and that you will recover if you follow the usual path addicts experience. Science tells us this. Understanding this truth allows you to maximize your opportunities to recover by clearing away the underbrush impeding your recovery.

CASE: Alan, at age thirty-five, had smoked since he was a teen. He had been reading up on research on brain images of drug users. He summed up what he had learned: "Smoking lights up the pleasure center of your brain. That's because nicotine activates the same reward pathways in the brain that other drugs of abuse like cocaine and amphetamines do. Research has shown that nicotine increases the levels of dopamine and adrenaline in the brain, neurochemicals that are responsible for feelings of pleasure and well-being. I can't produce enough of these chemicals anymore to feel okay without smoking, so I'd go through withdrawal if I stop smoking. I might never be able to experience pleasure again, in fact! How *could* I quit?"

Thinking Like an Addict

Here's the story: a way of thinking about addiction has grown up in the United States based on our temperance history. It is furthered by our modern "brain revolution," supposedly steeped in the biology of behavior and reinforced by an economic juggernaut, that purports to find in neuroscience a full and tidy explanation for addictive behavior. Unfortunately, these cultural beliefs bear little resemblance to the reality of addiction and are not just unhelpful—but detrimental—to people who develop addictions. This is because both the 12 steps and the "new" neuroscience strive to convince you that you are an addict and will always remain an addict, which, by and large, isn't true. And if you dispute any part of this story, you are in denial, proof positive of everything they say.

How can I say that the standard addiction treatment is detrimental? I can prove it. A study compared people trying to stay off cigarettes, having quit, with or without nicotine replacement therapy (NRT)—nicotine gum or patches.[1] The neuroscientific model of nicotine addiction is that addicts become so accustomed to having nicotine in their systems that to deplete their accustomed level of nicotine disrupts their bodies and minds, creating irresistible cravings that cause them to light up. It *is* true that smoking is a serious addiction; those experienced in multiple addictions place smoking at the top of the list of difficulty of quitting—alongside heroin, above cocaine, alcohol, and amphetamines.[2]

The quitting study, conducted by the most prestigious anti-tobacco group in the United States, the Center for Global Tobacco Control at

Harvard, tracked a group of eight hundred smokers trying to quit who either did or did not use gum or patches. The investigators found that those who used NRT to quit didn't do better than those who quit without it. In fact, the most dependent smokers—for whom NRT is supposed to be most helpful—were twice as likely to relapse to smoking if they relied on NRT than if they did not.

There were howls of outrage from NRT specialists. Here's a typical response from a professional in the field who read my *Huffington Post* story on the subject: "What this article tells us is what we already know: that simply providing the availability of over the counter NRT without the guidance and support of a trained tobacco treatment specialist is not very effective."[3] Except that's not what happened. "Odds of relapse were unaffected by use of NRT for 6 (or more) weeks either *with* or without professional counseling." The researchers who conducted the study were deeply invested in NRT. "We were hoping for a very different story," said Dr. Gregory N. Connolly, director of the Harvard Center.[4] These committed anti-tobacco warriors thus wasted millions of dollars—and years of effort.

How is it possible that such advanced medical technology for ending smoking is *more often than not* counterproductive? Certainly, some people succeed at *quitting*[5] with Nicorette gum or patches, and some remain tobacco free—but the bulk do not, and there are more productive treatment investments. The key to quitting an addiction is motivation, along with a belief in the possibility of succeeding—these factors are essential whether quitting addiction with, or without, treatment.[6] Those who depend on NRT believe both (1) that they can quit without the necessary personal commitment, and (2) that they *cannot* quit by means of their own personal strength and resources. In other words, they think like addicts—*which NRT forces them to do.* The moment of truth comes if and when these quitters also quit the nicotine replacement (which, of course, is addictive itself). *Most quickly relapse.*

What Is Addiction?

Addiction is not a by-product of the effects drugs have on your neurochemistry.[7] It is also not your inherited neurochemical destiny. Addiction is a reliance on an involvement to run interference for your experience of your internal and external worlds. Addiction is a normal part of human experience, as is recovery. Addiction occurs when a person seeks out an experience, ritual, or reward to the exclusion—and detriment—of all other goals and activities. The measure of addictiveness is how absorbing, compelling, and harmful to the person an involvement is. Nothing else matters.[8] Addiction can take the form of substance abuse or of compulsive behaviors like sex, gambling, or overeating. Whatever the involvement, to qualify as addictive it must lead to "significant impairment or distress." But it does occur on a sliding scale—yes, you can be more or less addicted.

The fifth edition of the American Psychiatric Association's *Diagnostic and Statistical Manual of Mental Disorders* (*DSM-5*), released in 2013, officially recognizes for the first time that addiction can occur with something other than drugs and alcohol—that "something" is gambling.[9] But we are all aware of many more addictions than drugs and alcohol. That food can be addictive—that people struggle against compulsive eating impulses that make them unhappy and harm them—is, seemingly all at once, being discovered by everybody. By a recent crop of neuro-diet doctors who claim that people become addicted to sugar/carbohydrates—that those foods light up the brain just as cocaine does,[10] by authors of popular memoirs,[11] and by analyses of American food production.[12] Another evident example is love addiction. I wrote *Love and Addiction* with Archie Brodsky in 1975 (in which we also discussed gambling and food addictions).[13] Since that time, the discovery that love and sex are addictive has been an expanding universe in American psychiatry and psychology, drawing in neuroscientists,[14] health writers,[15] and filmmakers[16] (the referenced sources are only a small reflection of their number).

Addiction is a response to life circumstances ranging from trauma to an inability to deal with everyday demands to being in a depressed-traumatic time in your life. It can be short-term and limited in time and place or a chronic pattern. The most important thing for you to know about addiction—knowledge the disease theory denies you—is that most people, sooner or later, naturally outgrow it. Research continually demonstrates this truth. For instance, the National Institute on Alcohol Abuse and Alcoholism (NIAAA) discovered through a massive national survey of Americans' drinking histories that 75 percent of alcohol-dependent people recover and that the large majority do it on their own, without treatment or AA.[17] The director of the research project, Dr. Mark Willenbring, noted: "It can be a chronic, relapsing disease. But it isn't usually."[18]

You don't need a study to tell you this about addiction. You have witnessed—or even experienced—this yourself: You must know someone who has quit smoking. Or maybe *you* have quit. As I noted above, smoking is certified by multi-substance addicts as among the most difficult drug addictions to overcome. Why has it been so hard—and still is for many—to accept that smoking is addictive in the same way as other drugs?[19] Because our very familiarity with the substance allows us to reject myths about it—although pharmaceutical companies and associated physicians still insist that you need their products and services to quit. Yet, even with such ubiquitous marketing, most people quit smoking on their own, without treatment, as they have always done.[20]

Here's a scenario that will make sense to you:

> Phil, who had begun smoking in his early teens, had tried to quit smoking numerous times in his life but had finally resigned himself to being "a smoker." In his late sixties, Phil awoke in a hospital bed after a heart attack. His first impulse was to light a cigarette. He asked his daughter, whose face he saw above him, to get him a cigarette and wheel him outside so that he could smoke. She told him that if he touched another cigarette, she would never speak to him again.
>
> Phil never smoked again.

How did Phil's experience relate to Alan's view of his addiction—a view pushed by the leading figures in the addiction field? They fundamentally contradict one another. Here's what happened for Phil. Phil's core life wasn't about being a smoker. When push came to shove, it turned out he was prepared to sacrifice smoking when it was counterweighted by what was most meaningful to him—being a father to his daughter. In fact, prioritizing parental love has cured more addictions than all other "methods" in the history of addiction combined—and will always do so.[21]

This isn't to say Phil did it easily—after all, he had been smoking for half a century—or that any smoker can or will quit quickly. But it doesn't help anyone to declare the task impossible! People may say, "I just can't live—be—without [smoking, drinking, pill taking . . .*]." It's a common

---

*Please be aware of and observe the cautions in quitting cold turkey reviewed in Chapter 3.

sentiment, one that you might share. The truth is, however, that the qualities that make you *you* are much more powerful and abiding than any addiction. When people overcome addiction, it's because they align their behavior with who they really are. When people recognize that something they are doing interferes with their deepest values or goals, they can leave destructive compulsions behind. It's a natural life process. Of course, there are many people whose natural recovery process needs a boost, and those are the people for whom The PERFECT Program is designed.

The PERFECT Program offers the information, guidance, and tools to ignite and accelerate your natural recovery process. It is supported by the best research in the field. If you have been through the recovery mill, or even if you are just a normal consumer of pop culture and pop science, you have been steeped in a heady concoction of misinformation and superstition about addiction, like the following primal addiction tale:

> I was always different from normal people. I was out of control, but I was in denial. When some horrible thing happened, I asked for help. I continued to fight the truth, but finally "let go" and admitted that I have a disease that I am powerless over. So, I stopped trying to run my own life; I turned my life and will over to a Higher Power. I am now "grateful in recovery," counting every sober day as a gift, because my disease is always growing and I could relapse at any time and end up dead.

This redemption narrative—or "drunkalog"—is part of our cultural landscape. It's also a good place to start unraveling the history of addiction recovery in America, because the whole fairytale is bundled in this neat little package. Before I explain where these ideas originated, let's unpack the mythology:

- **Myth:** Addicts are different from normal people, because they're fundamentally incapable of controlling themselves (anyone who can is not a "real" addict).
- **Myth:** Addicts can never be like other—normal—people.
- **Myth:** Recovery requires "hitting bottom"—a do-or-die scenario.
- **Myth:** Recovery is a blessing, bestowed by an entity outside oneself.
- **Myth:** Addicts are powerless and cannot trust themselves, even when abstinent.

- **Myth:** Addiction is always an incurable, progressive, fatal disease.
- **Myth:** Recovery is a one-day-at-a-time proposition that *must* include absolute abstinence and lifelong 12-step work.

You may believe that addiction is a disease that you are powerless over. You may also believe that recovery requires you to place your belief that you are an addict at the forefront of your consciousness at all times and that your addiction explains every dumb thing you have ever done. Maybe you believe that recovery is an unending, lifelong process, that it requires a spiritual awakening and perpetual maintenance, including total dedication to meetings and "quit anniversaries." Meanwhile, you must avoid normal people, social situations, and mouthwash containing alcohol. Finally, you may think that the disease of addiction progresses full force, despite long periods of abstinence. That means that, if you drink a beer after twenty years on the wagon starting as a teen, you'll fall right back into your addiction as if you had been drinking uncontrollably the whole time.

All of this has been updated in the guise of modern neuroscience conflating the AA ideology with brain chemistry. But none of it is true. When you apply these ideas to other addictions—like sex, love, shopping, gambling, the Internet—you can see them as laughable. Addiction experts seem incapable of dismissing the obvious inconsistencies and self-evident untruths of the disease model, even with the wide swath of research that has undermined it. But *you* must reject these ideas because, otherwise, they will keep you from outgrowing your addiction.

Think of this question, "Is love or food an addiction?" How can something that all healthy people do be addictive? Then someone tells you how obsessed they were with a lover, not being able to sleep, devoting every waking minute to worrying and lamenting first about the relationship, then about its breakup, while avoiding all other activities and relationships.[22] Or consider Mika Brzezinski, who admitted that she "has been battling a junk-food addiction since she was 13 years old. She has spent much of her adult life consumed with food, operating on a disastrous cycle of binge eating, purging, and over-exercising to maintain an impossibly skinny figure."[23] The truth about addiction is that food and love are addictive in the same sense that pain-killers (including heroin), cocaine, and alcohol are—they are addictive for some people in some situations or at some moments in their lives. Nothing is itself inherently addictive.

So how useful is it for you to consider that you have a disease and abstain from all contact with that experience? As I discuss in Chapter 3, of course you can't abstain from love and food. And, on the other hand, the success rate for disease-oriented, abstinence-obsessed 12-step treatment—along with its neurochemical equivalents—is not better, and may actually be worse, than not receiving treatment at all. I showed this above in the case of smoking. Research has likewise found significantly higher rates of relapse among alcoholics in AA than among alcoholics who go about quitting on their own[24] or who are treated with other methods.[25] If you believe that taking one drink is identical to having one hundred drinks and that you have a progressive disease that makes you powerless to control yourself, you won't just hop off the wagon—you will swan dive off it. Indeed, William Miller and his colleagues at the University of New Mexico tracked subjects following outpatient treatment for their drinking problems. The researchers found two primary factors predicted the likelihood of relapse—"lack of coping skills and *belief in the disease model of alcoholism*."[26]

Relying on the recovery-world idea of addiction—now cloaked in neuroscience—as an unconquerable disease instead of as part of normal experience has hurt us badly. As new brain discoveries uncover new addictions all the time, all presumably as uncontrollable as the original addictive diseases, we nonetheless congratulate ourselves on our modernity and medical progress. Yet we have no fewer addicts now than we did a century ago, and probably more, many more. Why, then, do we feel so confident that we have a handle on addiction, while our addictive problems expand endlessly?

Where Did the Disease Model Come From?

America has a temperance tradition. Carry A. Nation—the axe-wielding, saloon-busting zealot—is the best-known figure in the Temperance Movement, which was the engine powering the passage of national Prohibition in the United States in 1920. Temperance was—and is—a large part of our thinking. For us, Carry Nation may be the face of rigid sanctimony. But her conception of alcohol's impact on society arose from the wellsprings of American culture. Temperance resonates powerfully with attitudes that took hold in America in the nineteenth century, continued to grow in the twentieth, and are still expanding in the twenty-first. At the same time, they catch in many people's throats, as they did during Prohibition.[27] And they always will.

Temperance envisioned an epic battle between Good and Evil. On the eve of national Prohibition, in a national radio hook-up heard by millions, the Reverend Billy Sunday expressed the Temperance viewpoint:

> The reign of tears is over. The slums will soon be a memory. We will turn our prisons into factories and our jails into storehouses and corncribs. Men will walk upright now, women will smile and the children will laugh. Hell will forever be rent [split asunder].[28]

Billy Sunday's legacy in our lives is a tragedy. (Sunday's demonization of alcohol didn't work at home—while he himself lived a long life and was a moderate drinker before donning the cloth, his two sons died prematurely due to their alcoholism.) Our Temperance tradition has effectively nailed one of America's feet to the floor, and we have been marching in circles ever since. Addiction to legal and illegal drugs and alcohol certainly remains with us, and by all measures is increasing. The growth in addiction includes many new drugs unknown during Temperance and many things that weren't even imagined, or that at least weren't so effortlessly accessible so that their addictiveness wasn't as obvious as it is today (Internet pornography, games, and gambling, among others).

This moralism cum science that pervades addiction theory and practice (as Alan Marlatt so succinctly put it, "The disease model is the moral model in sheep's clothing") cripples us. Why should we saddle ourselves with ideas about substance use and addiction that plainly and simply don't work, and that actually hobble our ability to deal with them individually and as a society? On top of our quirky American outlooks and cultural inertia, we have added a multi-billion-dollar addiction treatment industry that aggressively maintains the status quo. Thousands of treatment facilities, addiction counselors, publishers, and "recovery landlords" (people who run sober living facilities) are financially dependent on the revolving door created by their staggering failures. Onto this juggernaut have been added the pharmaceutical industry's and addiction medicine's claims about addiction—primarily the claim that we are doomed without their products and services.[29]

AA treats addiction with an appeal for divine intervention. The emergent but hidden truth is that current disease approaches reflect the same magical thinking that inspired Temperance activists a century ago—our supposedly modern genetic and neuroscientific approaches are actually more of the same. The abject failure of Prohibition did not fundamentally change our approach to substance abuse. Instead, it shifted our point of attack. In place of a universal ban on drinking, alcohol was transformed from a public demon to the personal one of alcoholism. The battlefield is not the nation at large so much as it is the individual. Our view has shifted from the addict as a moral failure to the addict as a disease victim, although the two ideas remain inextricably similar. As the devil takes control of evil-doers, internal genetic and biological forces take control of addicts. It's not their fault but, underneath it all, these theories still blame addicts for their weakness.

The remnants of Temperance and Prohibition are everywhere evident in the United States—in dry counties and cities, state alcohol monopolies, and alcohol "blue laws."[30] Many people—including public health officials—still hold that alcohol is inherently "evil" or the equivalent view that it's a poison with inexorably bad health effects. This remains true even now that the *Dietary Guidelines for Americans* in 2010 noted strong evidence that regular, moderate drinkers live longer because alcohol reduces heart disease.[31] Of course, most Americans believe that cocaine, heroin, and methamphetamines are evil incarnate and that once people use these substances, or use them regularly, the drugs' effects make addiction, brain damage, and other destructive consequences inevitable. But as I have shown in my books from *Love and Addiction* on, and am now joined in proving by others like Columbia University psychopharmacologist Carl Hart, the effects of illicit drugs are sensationalized to confirm our cultural beliefs.[32] Hart's and my purpose isn't to encourage drug use; people evidently have plenty of motivation for that on their own. It is to locate and address the source of the problem where it exists—for Hart, this is especially in inner-city environments.

The Brain Revolution

Hasn't all of the prior discussion been rendered moot by stunning advances in brain science—haven't brain scans, MRIs, and PET scans located exactly where in the brain addiction takes place? Can't we *see* it there? The short answer is "No." There is no brain scan according to which a person can be said to be addicted, as opposed to showing the acute or chronic effects of cocaine or another drug or powerful experience. No one is diagnosed as "addicted" based on a brain scan. And no one ever will be.

Science is not science when it is handmaiden to mythology, received opinion, entrenched business and professional interests, and ongoing government policy and, *especially*, when it isn't effective in the realm it was designed to handle. Ergo, we have the modern era of addiction science and medicine, as represented in the newly minted (in 2011) American Board of Addiction Medicine (ABAM). According to the *New York Times*, in an article entitled "Rethinking Addiction's Roots, and Its Treatment," addiction has finally been resolved by neuroscience![33]

This is an old, old story. In fact, the science already tells us that addiction can never be resolved neurochemically, genetically, or biologically.[34] And everyone—even the neuroscientific experts who flack the new disease approach—knows that this is true, and that addiction is increasing and will continue to increase. Let's take a trip back over the decades to 1977, when a prominent neurologist, Richard Restak—the excitement catching in his throat—called the newly discovered neurochemicals, the endorphins, "a group of substances that hold out the promise of alleviating, or even eliminating, such age-old medical bugaboos as pain, drug addiction, and, among other mental illnesses, schizophrenia."[35]

What fruits have we reaped so far from the neurochemistry revolution? Have mental illness and addiction disappeared? Have they decreased? In fact, they've increased dramatically beginning almost exactly at the time those words appeared.[36]

As for genes, you have heard about the Human Genome Project, which mapped all of the chemical sequences on human DNA—the stuff that determines our biologically inherited selves. That mapping was completed on April 14, 2003. But there is still no gene for addiction. Although the Human Genome Project has provided a wealth of information, its bottom line is that single genes—or even groups of genes—*cannot account* for complex conditions, behaviors, and mental dispositions.[37]

Pleasure and brain scans

There is a voice of the new addictive brain revolution—it's the voice of Nora Volkow, head of the National Institute on Drug Abuse (NIDA), heard on *60 Minutes*, in the *New York Times*, and inside all of our heads. And that voice says, "Addiction is all about the dopamine."[38] According to Volkow, drugs operate through dopamine receptors in impacting the pleasure centers of the brain. Since drugs stimulate people's pleasure centers, the person's brain becomes dependent on drugs in order to achieve pleasure. Or, genetically, addicts are initially deficient in their dopamine production and processing and therefore require drugs to achieve the pleasure the rest of us experience normally.

Simple and appealing, right? And it's science to boot. But does it make sense? Do people get addicted to pleasure? Don't we all experience more or less pleasure from many different things? And doesn't how we react to that pleasure depend on a myriad of factors? Perhaps you think that cocaine is different, much more pleasurable. Recall my discussion earlier that experienced addicts find cigarettes harder to quit—more addicting—than cocaine. But you don't have to use drugs to stimulate your dopamine levels: Volkow and associates "have used PET scans to show that even when cocaine addicts merely watch videos of people using cocaine, dopamine levels increase." Researchers "demonstrate similar dopamine receptor derangements in the brains of drug addicts, compulsive gamblers and overeaters who are markedly obese."[39]

Volkow's brain revolution is headed into every serious area of our lives. Many activities stimulate the brain's pleasure centers. And, now, Volkow and others are saying these are addictive in the same way drugs are because they activate the same parts of the brain. I noted that the new edition of American psychiatry's bible, *DSM-5*, for the first time recognizes as addictive a non-drug-taking activity—gambling.[40] In addition, the DSM committee is contemplating adding gaming as an addiction. But why stop there? As the authors of *The Chemistry Between Us: Love, Sex and the Science of Attraction* make clear, "Dopamine is involved in reward and motivation for everything we do in life—whether we're eating good food, drinking good wine or interacting with our kids and family."[41]

So, we learn, these groups of people—drug addicts, compulsive eaters, and gamblers—respond with brain changes to seeing, even thinking about, their addictive activities. Does this really explain why people become addicted—ruining their lives and those of their families? Does everyone whose brain lights up due to using cocaine become addicted, and do those who do stay addicted? Maybe they will become more restrained as they mature. Maybe they will occupy themselves with other things—leading more productive lives, doing the right thing, taking responsibility for the well-being of children—that will cause them to restrain themselves, as love of a child did for Rose and Phil.

If so many things stimulate dopamine production and the pleasure parts of the brain, and since all of us eat, have sex, and at some time were exposed to gambling or gaming (another activity to which many become addicted),[42] are we all addicted to one thing or another at some point? Perhaps we are. Then what might once have been considered human frailties to be worked on, alleviated, and perhaps even accepted become lifelong disease diagnoses. But, of course, we recognize that some people become addicted to the same activities while others do not. What, then, accounts for these individual differences?

Self-control and the brain

Can we locate addiction in the brain? Dopamine implicates the limbic system. But in addition to finding pleasure centers, neuroscientists must add another layer when they talk about addiction. These scientists recognize what you and I do—that not all people who experience pleasure from doing something, even very intense pleasure (think sex again, or eating), simply go out and repeat that activity ad infinitum. For instance, many people consume cocaine without being addicted to it—even though they, too, find it very pleasurable.[43] You know this is true, too, because people may become addicted to amphetamines in the same way they do to cocaine (remember Rose), and yet amphetamines are used in popular prescription drugs such as Adderall.

Why don't most become addicted? Addiction theorists focus on the frontal lobes as the center of "executive" control functions:

> Alcohol and substance abuse disorders involve continued use of substances despite negative consequences, i.e., loss of behavioral control of drug use. The frontal cortical areas of brain oversee behavioral control through executive functions. Executive functions include abstract

> thinking, motivation, planning, attention to tasks and inhibition of impulsive responses. Impulsiveness generally refers to premature, unduly risky, poorly conceived actions. Dysfunctional impulsivity includes deficits in attention, lack of reflection and/or insensitivity to consequences, all of which occur in addiction.[44]

And so addicts are marked by impulsivity, which is associated with the frontal lobes.

As with all such claims, this one involves a simplified and schematic idea of the brain. Figure 1 in the quoted reference is titled "A Simplified Schematic of Frontal Cortical and Limbic Brain Region Circuitry That Contribute to Addictive Behavior." You and I couldn't make sense of this "simplified" schematic, let alone the actually functioning brain, whose activities defy description. The limbic system is very, very complex and is associated with, among other things, emotions, pleasure, and memory. But Joseph LeDoux and many other neuroscientists regard it as impossible to map specific human experiences onto designated places in the brain—so many parts are involved in so many functions.[45] For LeDoux, this thinking traces back to ideas about brain anatomy that neuroscientists now know are inaccurate and no longer use. Do you remember phrenology?

In 2012, a study in the prestigious scientific journal, *Science*, reported finding a neurogenetic basis for substance abuse. The *Time* headline about the study read, "Siblings Brain Study Sheds Light on Roots of Addiction."[46] Subjects were identified based on their chronic use of various drugs: most often cocaine, but also amphetamines, heroin, and alcohol. These individuals were compared with their siblings, who weren't substance abusers. Presented with cognitive tests, both the chronic substance abusers and their non-abusing siblings showed poor impulse control compared with most people. "Brain scans also showed that siblings had similar abnormalities in the connections between their inferior frontal gyrus, an area of the brain involved with self-control."

Now, the question is, why did half the siblings become addicts if all were poor at controlling their impulses? Apparently not only were the drugs not responsible for addiction, but neither were the siblings' brain deficits, which the sibling subjects shared. What we still don't know from this study is why the siblings with similar brain structures and weak self-control differed in their substance abuse. Apparently, people don't control themselves or fail to do so solely because of the "connections between their inferior frontal gyrus."

The insightful author of the *Time* article, Maia Szalavitz, wrote:

> Interestingly, the authors note, these connectivity problems are similar to those seen in the brains of teenagers, a group that is characterized by impulsive behavior. It is almost as if the brains of addicts are less mature. Perhaps that helps explain why some addiction wanes with age. Studies find that most people who struggle with alcohol and other drugs in their 20s "are out" of their problems by their 30s, typically without treatment.

But if this impulsiveness/addictiveness is naturally outgrown, then why talk about a lifelong disease? We're in an entirely different realm altogether, the realm of *Recover!*.

Can people control themselves—how?

At the beginning of this chapter, I wrote that addiction is a consuming behavior or involvement that you rely on, but that detracts from your life by making you miserable or limiting your ability to engage the world freely and effectively. How does that fit with modern neuroscientific discoveries, such as that drugs and some experiences activate the limbic system and cause the body to produce pleasurable brain chemicals, such as dopamine? The body and brain thus become accustomed—acclimated—to this stimulation and production, and *can't live without it.*

Of course, that last phrase is the key. Alan figures he can't live without cigarettes stimulating his limbic system and producing dopamine; Phil seemingly acted that way—until he quit for his daughter's love. In fact, that drugs and gambling and shopping—and, as we have seen, not only these things—cause brain and neurochemical changes is really no great revelation. *Every* stimulus and human experience translates to some action of the brain. And the more powerful and engaging for you the experience, the greater the brain changes are likely to be. In this sense, then, *you* control your brain's reaction through how strongly you respond to something or how appealing you find it to be.

Your brain and neurological system adapt to this stimulation. Remember homeostasis in tenth-grade biology? The body, down to the cellular level, responds to stimulation by retracting its natural responses and creating counteracting responses, to achieve balance. You become inured to an experience, less sensitive to the stimuli, so that you need more of the external stimulation to achieve the same level of that experience that you initially attained with less effort. If that stimulation stops, the body springs back the opposite way, the more so as our body acclimates to the initial stimulus. Here is the neuroscience of all pleasure-addictions from Nora Volkow: "*Once the brain becomes less sensitive to dopamine, it 'becomes less sensitive to natural reinforcers' such as the 'pleasure of seeing a friend, watching a movie, or the curiosity that drives exploration.'*"[47] Volkow's definition of addiction here is actually quite close to mine, but for its being couched entirely in terms of your nervous system.

What is the most stimulating, pleasurable experience humans can have? For most, the answer is sex. The psychiatric diagnostic manual hasn't quite gotten around to recognizing sex as addictive. *DSM-5* also rejected *hypersexual disorder*, which sounds a lot like sexual addiction (not to mention the now-discredited *nymphomania*). It is defined by "evidence of personal distress caused by the sexual behaviors that interfere with relationships, work or other important aspects of life."[48] Yet it turns out that people with hypersexuality don't find sex any more stimulating—"They look just like normal people with high sex drive."[49]

Most of us—even with high sex drives—fit sex into the normal course of our lives, as pleasure subordinated to the rest of our needs, like making a living, raising children, fitting in with society, avoiding being classified as a sexual predator, and so on. Most of us control our sexual urges much of the time—although many of us have had our moments of uncontrollable delight, and misery, around sex and its deprivation. We wouldn't rape someone, kill for it, spend ourselves into insolvency, or otherwise ruin the rest of our lives to satisfy that itch in our loins. *This has always been true; it will always be true; nothing discovered in the brain can change this reality.*

Except now the advent of free Internet porn has led to a remarkably large number of addictions.[50] We all become used to—sated with—sex with the same partner. Most of us accept this—more or less. Sexual and marital best-sellers, marriage manuals, and *Cosmopolitan* are full of methods for keeping sexual desire alive and for restimulating couples' sex lives. Others remedy the loss of desire within long-term relationships by seeking the stimulation that comes with extramarital sex. Do those people experience more pleasure from sex, more satiation from long-term relationships, have deficient (or excessive) dopamine levels, or have bad inferior frontal gyru connections? Or are they just more likely to have extramarital affairs, for one reason or another?

Sexual addictions often take the form of addiction to Internet porn: "*I sold porn on the Internet for over 10 years. It ruined relationships and led me down a dark road of heavy use.*" Marnia Robinson (who writes a *Psychology Today* blog alongside mine) has focused on Internet porn and addiction, finding it the dominant addictive problem of our time. She describes men who masturbate throughout the day, lose the ability to engage in normal sex with, or be aroused by, spouses and other lovers, and become slaves to porn.

Can no one then overcome an addiction to porn? Of course they can. The above quotes come from a blogpost by Robinson and Gary Wilson called: "Guys Who Gave Up Porn."[51] Here's what happens to them:

> Most experience weeks of uncomfortable, temporary withdrawal symptoms [note from me: withdrawal symptoms *are* temporary—that's the definition of withdrawal], such as mood swings (irritability, anxiety, despair, apathy, restlessness), insomnia, fatigue, very frequent urination, intense cravings or flat libido, etc. One man charted his ups and downs. Happily, recovering users often become more responsive to pleasure even before the withdrawal symptoms and hypersensitivity to porn cues stop: *After 34 days I tested myself. I could masturbate to orgasm without thinking about anything for the first time of my life. And erections came much more frequently and stronger. At the same time I knew with absolute certainty that the process wasn't finished yet.*

How and why do people stop being addicted?

I've used the term "neuromeme" to mean the style of representing human experience, motivation, and behavior in neurological—brain chemistry and mechanics—terms and images. As a culture, we increasingly seek explanations for our behavior in neurochemicals and brain activation, as though that were the total answer. The most important part of this neuromeme, I have shown, is the idea that we have no control over whether and how the addictive process starts and, once it's occurred, whether or not we quit. This is the "hijacked brain" invented by Volkow's predecessor as NIDA director, Alan Leshner[52] (and popularized by Bill Moyers's

1998 PBS series, *Close to Home: Moyers on Addiction*, on which I was a consultant).[53]

These neuromemes are repeated constantly in popular broadcast media, magazines, and Internet sites. We now as a culture think in these terms. Yet nothing in those PET scans indicates that something has happened to a person's brain to finally hijack it, the exact moment this happens, and when it stops—which, as we shall see, is the typical outcome for addicts.

One addict who personifies this mystery—how the brain is apparently hijacked, but then recovers—is Marc Lewis, who writes about his life as a drug addict in *Memoirs of an Addicted Brain: A Neuroscientist Examines His Former Life on Drugs* (Perseus, 2011). Lewis is a neuroscientist. He quit his drug addiction. Here's what Lewis says about that:

> So this time was obviously hugely different. How did it work? I'm really not sure. Basically, I reported what happened. The details are accurate. I didn't have an instruction manual, so I can't really say what was going on or precisely what I did that time that unlocked a new door. But here, I'll try. I had recently endured two particularly shitty events. My girlfriend left me, which broke my heart, and my friends found me, semi-comatose, on a toilet seat in a public building with a needle sticking out of my arm, which was intensely shame-inducing. I think by then I had built up a lot of rage, not just self-contempt and all that but real rage—toward drugs.[54]

A lot like Rose and Phil, really, when you think about it—love and physical illness and shame caused both of them to quit their addictions. All three of them, including Lewis, were addicted, and thought they were stuck. But events proved them wrong.

Lewis deals with what we would all agree was the most important part of his addiction—quitting it—as almost an afterthought, as reflected in his title for the piece: "How I Quit. . . . At Least, How I Think I Quit." Lewis says he didn't have the manual for brain change—even though he is a neuroscientist and his book is full of discussions of the brain. But, really, at its base, Lewis's book is about his awkward and isolated growing up and the relief that drugs provided him. What he is really doing is trying to translate experiential psychology into neuroscience. That actually can't be done—as Lewis finds: despair, love, and shame just don't come stamped with labels on brain scans. Experience and brain dynamics remain forever distinct entities.

Moreover, as Carl Hart and Maia Szalavitz note about media images of permanent drug-induced brain damage in the case of methamphetamines,

> The problem is that the hype may do serious damage to those struggling with methamphetamine problems. "One of the major reasons I did the review is that one of the most effective treatments is cognitive behavioral therapy," says Hart. "The argument has been made that these people can't benefit because they are cognitively impaired and can't pay attention. There's no scientific evidence to support that position."
>
> Indeed, the idea that those who take methamphetamine are more likely to fail at treatment or need longer-term care than people with other addictions is not supported by the data, either. Unfortunately, by pushing the idea that methamphetamine damages the brain, researchers may inadvertently deter treatment seeking, both by making people with addictions feel hopeless and by making providers have less faith in their ability to help.[55]

Of course, treatment may consist of convincing addicts of exactly these myths, which is one reason Rose felt she had to reject the treatment she was offered in order to recover.

The abuse trap

Lewis's painful upbringing and subsequent drug abuse are not unusual—although, as we will see, his experience is far from the typical substance abuser's or addict's case. But the abuse explanation has become another prominent theme in the addiction lexicon, and many unwary addicts have dead-ended on this sidetrack. Let me note without hesitation that childhood abuse is bad for human beings and produces bad outcomes. But, in the overwhelming majority of cases, it is surmountable and people do overcome it. Nonetheless, there is now an entire subcontinent of addiction clinicians who seek out unremembered childhood abuse as the explanation for every case of addiction they encounter. Moreover, many trace back such re-imagined abuse to imagined brain chemistry. Even such a prominent addiction specialist as Gabor Maté, the Canadian physician and author of *In the Realm of Hungry Ghosts*, believes that early abuse, neglect, and even—casting a wide net—stress and lack of affection permanently impair people's ability to process brain chemicals that provide us with pleasure and pain relief.

Maté then claims these deficiencies in addicts' neurosystems cause them to self-medicate to replace their missing neurostimulation. This is actually a specialized version of the brain/neurochemical model we saw, but now steeped in childhood abuse, in which people are addicted to drugs as replacements for missing brain chemicals brought on by the abuse. As important as is Maté's work with addicts, his simplistic vision of addiction in which abuse history and imagined biochemical changes become the essential causes of people's self-destructive behavior can be as incapacitating as genetic neurochemical deficiency models.

It is not enough to say that this model is highly conjectural. It also isn't true—that is, it makes little sense of the world. A huge epidemiological study of early childhood experiences found that 3.5 percent of people with four or more adverse childhood experiences ever injected drugs.[56] It was a higher number than for the general population, but still only a tiny portion of the group. Of course, few people in the overall population become heroin addicts, but the same research included alcohol dependence. With drinking as with drugs, the rates of dependence follow the same elevated trajectory depending on the number of adverse childhood experiences. But they are still only slightly higher for abuse victims—16 percent versus around 10 percent. So abuse models of addiction like Maté's tell us little. And even when abuse victims become addicts, there is no way to separate out negative psychological consequences of their dysfunctional upbringings. These consequences, even though they can't be translated into identifiable brain malfunctions, could nonetheless fuel a person's addiction.

Worst of all, focusing on childhood as the determinant of addiction detracts from our awareness of people's natural tendency to overcome abuse and addictive experiences. We might ask, first, what protects the other 96.5 percent of abuse sufferers who don't inject drugs and the 84 percent who do not become alcohol dependent? On top of this, what about the strong tendency described throughout this chapter and *Recover!* for people with addictions to recover naturally? Focusing on abuse as an irreversible cause of your addiction does not support your efforts to confront your abuse and overcome its effects on your life.

CASE: Suzanna was a doctoral student, age twenty-seven, who—it might seem ironic—worked with an alcohol research group. Ironic because she worried about her drinking. She drank daily—rarely becoming intoxicated—but needing to have three to four drinks of alcohol to feel okay, and sometimes on weekends drinking more. She felt guilty about her drinking and didn't let other people know about it. Reading writers like Marc Lewis, the neuroscientist quoted above, she decided her drinking was permanently lodged in her brain due to her childhood experience. For Suzanna had been abandoned by her mother.

Suzanna, like many modern Americans, seeks an answer to her problems in a childhood that her reading tells her has irreversibly altered her brain. How *helpful* is that for her? There will never be—never can be—a way to find lesions in the brain that stand for Suzanna's abandonment, ones that could clearly point to her drinking issues. And, please do recall, Lewis himself overcame his drug-injection addiction, more or less spontaneously. But Suzanna was caught up in this sidetrack, to the exclusion of those avenues she might have pursued successfully.

Your brain changes when you change

Neuroscience doesn't explain addiction nearly as well as it explains recovery. This is because neuroscience has the most to say about the brain's ability to be reshaped—and to reshape itself—while forming new connections, which is called *neuroplasticity*. Researchers time and again have discovered how adaptable the brain is—for example, brain-injured people typically replace lost functioning by shifting these functions to other parts of the brain ("rewiring") and through new neural development.[57] People's brains change all the time due to external and internal stimuli. *All* of the various experiences you have compete, counteract, and disallow one another. Most important, you control which of these experiences are seminal or dominant, as when Phil (or anyone) quits smoking because his values override a mindless habit.

Now that brain chemistry has become a runaway train, serious writers and clinicians believe they must point at their brains and talk in neurospeak when discussing every kind of behavior. In their brilliant book, *Brainwashed: The Seductive Appeal of Mindless Neuroscience* (Basic Books, 2013), Sally Satel and Scott Lilienfeld detail the extent to which neuroscientific theories pervade modern thinking. Calling this the "neurocentric" view of the mind, Satel and Lilienfeld detail how this view is based on simplistic and inaccurate ideas about what brain scans can actually tell us. At the same time, they show that this view denies the reality of choice and personal responsibility and leads to bad decision making throughout society, including not only psychiatry, but also the legal system.

Obviously, the same reliance on brain concepts and neuromemes is occurring in the addiction field. High-end practitioners use brain scans or similar tests to show that individuals' frontal lobes aren't sufficiently activated. What is sufficient frontal lobe activity, how complex neural patterns in the prefrontal cortex in combination with other parts of the brain express themselves in thinking and behavior, whether drug takers who use and don't become addicted show similar MRI results—all those considerations are irrelevant to these practitioners. It is a way of thinking people often want to hear. The crucial difference is between those, like Dr. Drew of "Celebrity Rehab,"[58] who claim that "hypofrontalism" is a permanent brain disease that means people's self-restraint is dead and can't be revived and those who understand that self-restraint is an area for addicts to work on using cognitive-behavioral techniques.

People may find it useful to think in terms of their brains when they change old patterns.[59] But you don't need to see a brain graphic to know that people initiate change. Because you know people like Phil and Rose, and you may be one of those people, who quit smoking or other addictions. The "hijacked brain" and "chronic brain disease" memes ignore this natural ability of the brain to reform itself. The idea that a person's brain scan depicts their addictive past, present, and future is poppycock.

Some of the ways to change brain function that have been measured include meditation and through related mindfulness, breathing, and relaxation techniques and self-acceptance.[60] One way to think of mindfulness practices to defeat craving is that they disconnect existing brain patterns, what some call the neural craving network, while creating new neural pathways.[61] But your principal concerns are the practices that you consciously control—the more often you engage in such techniques, the more readily your brain adapts and responds to them. What is critical is to start, practice, and continue these new ways of thinking and acting.

Working against people's own natural growth

As I have indicated, AA and the 12 steps are popular out of all relation to their ability to address and to remedy addiction. But, nowadays, the public relations behemoth in support of chronic brain disease-ology has even more backing than from celebrity recovering addicts/alcoholics who promote the 12 steps. Many more institutions, livelihoods, and reputations depend on the disease of addiction today than when Bill Wilson and Bob Smith reached into American religious mythology to create the 12-step philosophy. These include now addiction medicine, manufacturers of an emerging array of pharmaceuticals, and the neuroscientific research industry itself, all in addition to the vast network of Betty Ford–style, 12-step rehabs.[62] Only, now, the usual 12-step bromides and treatment are couched in neurochemical and brain terms while simply performing the same ancient rituals based on the same faulty logic, data, and visions of the sources and trajectory of most addiction. This large—and growing—industry requires that more of us believe that we are suffering from lifelong addictive diseases. What is happening to the idea that we can outgrow, that we can be encouraged to outgrow, and that we should outgrow addiction?

Outgrowing addiction

The ability to change an addiction is something we all know about. As in Maia Szalavitz's analysis of the decline in impulsivity as people mature (and maybe experience changes to their inferior frontal gyrus), we have all seen and experienced it. When interviewing sociologist Thomas Vander Ven, who, in his book *Getting Wasted*, described how most college binge drinkers (more than 40 percent of undergraduate students) are drinking to overcome social anxieties and to gain a sense of belonging in their first time living away from home,[63] an interviewer for the online magazine *Salon* had an affecting reaction:

> A lot of what you say really rings true. I definitely had a lot of social anxiety when I was in college. I was on a varsity rowing team, and I was gay, and I drank partly to get over the awkwardness that came with that. . . . And as soon as I left college—it was almost instantaneous—the idea of being hungover just became extraordinarily unappealing and I stopped drinking so much.

Vander Ven responded to his young interviewer: "That's a lot of people's experience—drinking in college is just a very different enterprise than once you graduate." That is, unless you are convinced you have a lifelong disease. In the meantime, Hazelden and other treatment providers are expanding big-time into treatment facilities dedicated to adolescents—in the case of Hazelden, to the tune of a new multi-million-dollar campus for teens.[64]

Why don't we hear from all of the people who outgrow their alcoholic/addictive phases? On the one hand, it's so natural that we don't find it exceptional or noteworthy—even as Hazelden and others hard-sell the opposite, counterintuitive idea. For example, now that Angelina Jolie is a transcendent movie star, world-moving humanitarian, mother, and role model,[65] who focuses on her troubled youth, when she was suicidally depressed, cut herself, and used heroin along with other drugs?[66] Or, do you remember now that Drew Barrymore appeared on the cover of *People* in 1989 (January 16), age thirteen, as America's youngest addict? She had been in rehab and confessed, "I'm Drew, and I'm an addict-alcoholic," and that now she was embarked on recovery. She subsequently relapsed, attempted suicide, and reentered rehab, as she described in her 1990 memoir, *Little Girl Lost*, published when she was fifteen.

The *People* article included an analysis by a psychiatrist and adolescent addiction expert, Dr. Derek Miller: "Although there is nothing available clinically to test for genetic dependence," Dr. Miller admitted, "parents should be very careful to keep their children off of all alcohol if there is a history of either alcoholism or biologically based depression in the family." In other words, Drew inherited her alcoholism-addiction from her substance-abusing parents and forebears (like grandfather John Barrymore). Miller continued: "Abstinence is the key to all treatment." Although, he added, "the younger the adolescent, the harder it is for them to understand they have a problem." You know, the problem that they were born addicts-alcoholics, a destiny they can never escape.

Flash forward to 2012, when Barrymore once again appeared in *People* (June 4), with the announcement: "Drew Barrymore: She's a Vintner!," one who had "lots of knowledge and was passionate about her wine." But everyone is so aware—it is so obvious—that most people successfully outgrow their youthful substance abuse that no one cares to reflect back to the earlier *People* treatises on Drew and addiction to reevaluate their ideas about alcoholism and other addictions. Do you think Dr. Miller has greatly revised his theories based on his monumental miscalculations about Drew? Not likely. Believing the disease theory of addiction means never having to say you're sorry—just as no one worries about a few miscalculations about how the discovery of endorphins and a special alcoholism gene would soon end addiction and solve alcoholism, or about how nicotine replacement holds the key to quitting smoking addiction, even though it actually fosters it.

Change, Change, Change

CASE: Dori had been drinking alcoholically for twenty years, since her early teens. Most nights of her life she fell asleep in a drunken blackout. She also smoked for all that time. If anyone were a candidate for permanent, debilitating alcoholism, it was Dori. She had been in and out of 12-step programs her entire life, as well as psychiatric treatment. Nothing had changed for her.

Dori was extremely concerned about her appearance—she always dressed well, exercised, and was hyperconscious about her weight and diet. One night, Dori walked into a bar and stared at several women arrayed along the bar's counter. In the harsh light of the place, Dori—already a little bit drunk—saw herself in the row of run-down women. Dori quit drinking that night. And smoking. And psychiatric meds. She had a rough several weeks dealing with the upheavals in her system that withdrawal caused. But more important for her to deal with was the giant empty space at the core of her life that alcohol had filled for more than half of that life. Yet recovery proved to be enduring for Dori.

The truth, and how to harness it for your recovery

Not only must you reject the fear-mongering addiction madness of the last century, brought up-to-date by Dr. Drew, the American Society of Addiction Medicine, and neuromemes—you can replace it with a sane, empowering understanding based on principles grounded in reality. A truly human view of addiction accepts that a wide range of factors contribute to the development of addiction. But what most concern you—what offer you the best chances in life—are those factors that you can address and change. You stop being addicted by expanding your psychological horizons, creating new interests, and maturing (remember, Nora Volkow characterized addiction as when people lose the "pleasure of seeing a friend, watching a movie, or the curiosity that drives exploration") and by focusing on your values, working on skills you need to improve your life, and developing larger purposes.

Remember our list of myths about addiction? Let's replace them with these essential truths, and explore each in turn.

- Addiction and recovery are common—typical—in human experience.
- Addiction, by its nature, is artificial and, therefore, can be overcome.
- You have the resources within you to overcome addiction, completely, forever.
- There is nothing and no one more able than you to begin and sustain your recovery.

Addiction and recovery are common—typical—in human experience

Are Angelina Jolie, Drew Barrymore, and Dr. Adi Jaffe (a therapist who Dr. Drew claims couldn't have been really addicted since he now drinks moderately after a major amphetamine addiction[67]) the only people who have come down from addiction to become moderate substance users? In fact, they are in the majority. As I wrote at the beginning of this chapter, the National Institute on Alcohol Abuse and Alcoholism has conducted a giant survey of Americans' drinking lives. This study is called NESARC (National Epidemiologic Survey on Alcohol and Related Conditions). NESARC interviewed more than 43,000 representative Americans eighteen and older about their lifetime of drinking—interviews were conducted in 2001–2002 and a second wave in 2004–2005.

About one in ten Americans qualified for a diagnosis of alcoholism at some point in their lives, the government's alcoholism researchers determined. Here's what happened to them:[68] "Twenty years after onset of alcohol dependence, about three-fourths of individuals are in full recovery; more than half of those who have fully recovered drink at low-risk levels without symptoms of dependence. . . . Only 13 percent of people with alcohol dependence ever receive specialty alcohol treatment" (this includes attending AA). And no higher a percentage of treated than of untreated alcoholics recover (28 percent of treated alcoholics are currently alcoholic, compared with 24 percent of the untreated)![69] These untreated alcoholics are the invisible Americans we *don't* hear about because they violate most Americans' beliefs. But, unless the United States is wasting a fortune utilizing its best researchers and interviewers,[70] most people overcome alcoholism themselves, as they do smoking and every other addiction.

Perhaps, you feel, drug addiction is very different from alcoholism and smoking. According to NESARC, which also measured drug abuse, it is. *Drug addicts more readily give up their addictions than do alcoholics and smokers*! NESARC reports, "26 years after first becoming dependent, half the people at some time dependent on nicotine were in remission, a milestone reached for alcohol after 14 years, for cannabis six years, and for cocaine five years." Although there were not enough heroin addicts in this population to analyze, the investigators found that other data showed their remission point likewise to be quicker than for alcohol and cigarettes.[71] In other words, Rose's relatively quick recovery from her meth addiction and Phil's lengthy effort to quit cigarettes, with Dori in between, are typical. The reason, as Rose's case shows, is that it is harder to maintain an illicit-drug lifestyle.

Another study of the NESARC data found that 80 percent of people who had been dependent on an illegal drug were in recovery. Moreover, investigator Gene Heyman showed, "no matter how long ago someone became dependent on an illegal drug or alcohol, their chances of achieving remission remain the same." Heyman thus emphasized that, contrary to AA's idea of addiction as a progressive disease—or claims that neurochemical changes fix an addiction permanently in the brain—people are just as likely to quit at any point in their addiction career. Heyman found that addicts quit at the point when they can finally realize their values and aspirations.

These analyses of the drug addiction data from NESARC were summarized in an issue of the *Effectiveness Bank Bulletin*. This issue labeled a third large study "**Recovery is the norm**," in which the renowned alcoholism scholar William White synthesized the results of hundreds of studies of drug addicts and alcoholics: "Recovery is not an aberration achieved by a small and morally enlightened minority of addicted people. If there is a natural developmental momentum within the course of these problems, it is toward remission and recovery." What a powerful message this is, if only it were broadcast as loudly as is the one that addiction is embedded in our brains and our lives, presumably forever for most people. But such recovery from drug addiction goes unrecognized, as it does with alcoholism, because it usually occurs without treatment.

Nonetheless, most people understand—or at least live out—this message for themselves. Another massive study of drug abuse, the National Survey on Drug Use and Health, is conducted annually by the Substance Abuse and Mental Health Services Administration. Here are the figures for abuse of, or dependence on, either alcohol or drugs by age group for 2011 (these figures remain essentially the same year after year)[72]:

TABLE 2.1 **Percentage of Americans Who Abuse or Are Dependent on Drugs or Alcohol for Each Age Group**

Age Group	*% Abuse or Dependent*
18–19	17
20–22	20
23–25	17
26–29	13
30–34	12
35–49	8
50–59	5
60+	3

We see again from government data that substance abuse is a common trait among the young, but that large numbers of people cease their abuse and dependence after their early twenties. Twenty percent (one in five) of those at this age are clinically diagnosable as either abusing or dependent on alcohol or drugs, compared with 12 percent in their early thirties, and down to 5 percent in their fifties.

ENVIRONMENTS THAT ENCOURAGE—OR DISCOURAGE—ADDICTION

There are many scenarios in which people are rendered unable to cope. Some people are thrust into traumatic situations that are beyond anyone's ability to control, and some people simply do not have the skills to manage their obligations and the vagaries of everyday life, at least for the time being. Whether they are having trouble navigating traumatic circumstances like war or abuse or simply having difficulties in daily coping, people may seek a ready escape in mind-altering substances and other addictions. And, once they have turned to addictive remedies, the possibility of regaining control of their lives can seem even more remote.

History has provided the example of addicted Vietnam GIs.[73] Heroin use was rampant among American soldiers in Vietnam, where the drug was readily available. Among those addicted in Vietnam, only a fraction (one in eight, or 12 percent) became re-addicted stateside. This was true even though *half* tried a narcotic when they returned.[74] What explains this? Turning to and relying on a powerful analgesic to relieve stress made sense in Vietnam, but not afterwards. As Vietnam fades into history, we can still readily discern the powerful addictive urges produced when normal routes to escape and advancement are blocked in our inner cities. But it is no more permanent a condition there than it was for most veterans when they returned to manageable environments.

Vietnam demonstrated that addiction doesn't define a person, that being able to gain satisfaction through engagement with the world trumps addiction. There is no better "treatment." The Vietnam heroin experience showed us the recipe for recovery: people avoid and overcome addiction when they have positive options, meaningful goals, and control of their lives.

Addiction, by its nature, is artificial and, therefore, can be overcome

Like the soldiers who depended on heroin to release them from horrific circumstances that they could not change, addicted people seek refuge in any powerful, consuming experience that allows them to cope with a life that feels meaningless or out of control—a feeling that is both worsened and relieved by their addiction. The addiction further fills countless hours beyond those eaten up in altered states of consciousness or compulsions. Think of all the mental and emotional energy an addiction wastes: days planned around purchasing and consuming the substance or practicing the activity; fielding negative fallout (like angry co-workers, family members, and friends; mounting bills; health problems); making solemn promises to stop; remorse and guilt.

Yet, as painful and self-defeating as these feelings are, their predictability sustains addicts and even lends a bizarre sense of purpose to their lives. Rather than being a medical mystery, *addiction makes complete psychological sense.* It's a natural human response to unmanageable life circumstances, one through which people mistakenly attempt to find purpose and a sense of well-being. They're wrong, of course, and can't succeed at it. But this is more of a perverted effort to balance one's life than a permanent addicted place in your brain. *Addiction is not who people are.* And most people figure this out as they go along, because—contrary to claims of denial—it's not that hard to figure out. People perceive the mounting negative consequences for their lives and, if given half a chance, they clamber out of the addiction. We have seen through the best, most comprehensive research about people's real lives that this is what happens for most people, and not only Vietnam vets.[75]

You have the resources within you to overcome addiction, completely, forever

When I point out that people recover without treatment, this of course doesn't mean they didn't get help, or that people recover completely on their own. They rely on community, family, personal resources. Thus, becoming connected with others is one of the best predictors that you will recover. Likewise, as I will show in succeeding chapters, everything you bring to the effort—your knowledge, education, work skills, values, commitments, friends, family, community involvements, interests, health—offers a helpful boost. And, so, along with the types of therapy that can be helpful, along with the passage of time and maturity, any resource you possess aids in achieving your own, true-to-yourself recovery. And any of these assets you acquire or improve as you work for recovery will contribute to achieving it.

So, we see that people have the wherewithal, or can gain it, to overcome addiction for themselves—you included. Why do they recover? You know what happens: people settle down emotionally, they develop responsibilities—work, children, financial obligations—the usual. It comes with the human territory of growing up or, in addiction terms, "maturing out." You may have failed to mature out when you might have had the chance. You may even have developed your addiction later, after supposed maturity, even—unfortunately—as a parent (like Rose). Perhaps you lacked the necessary skills or emotional resources that come to most people in adulthood. But that's water under the bridge. The PERFECT Program is your second chance—your second emergence into maturity.

EFFECTIVE TREATMENT

Research also shows you the best way to get help to help yourself. Should you seek or need treatment, or even if you just want to learn what sorts of treatments work so that you can use their best elements, we turn to research on *evidence-based treatment*. Psychological investigators have repeatedly found evidence for the effectiveness of therapies steeped in real human functioning. Researchers have performed a series of meta-analyses, which combine results from all investigations of treatment effectiveness. One such comprehensive analysis ranked 12-step therapy and AA thirty-seventh and thirty-eighth among forty-eight possible treatment options.[76] More critically, combining the results of several such analyses, these addiction therapies are the five steady winners[77]:

- Cognitive-behavioral therapy
- Community reinforcement approach
- Motivational interviewing
- Relapse prevention (which is also cognitive-behavioral)
- Social skills training

All of these effective treatments approach addiction as ingrained behaviors and habits of mind, fostered by life situations. Although people with even the most intense addictions—like Dori—may ultimately solve their addictions for themselves, others—including you—may seek and benefit from effective treatment (unlike all of the programs Dori went through). What you find is that the evidence-based treatments in this list all reject the notion of an incurable disease and instead harness and fortify people's own resources. They fuel people's motivation to quit, counteract or change their environment, rely on their social community, and develop their life skills. And all *create a sense of personal empowerment.* That's what *you* need to do.

Along with this research on effective treatments comes mindfulness research. Mindfulness is learning to be aware of your thoughts and impulses, to stand outside of them in order to gain control of them. The thoughts might be there (along with urges, cravings, compulsions), but you learn that you do not have to let them lead you. Mindfulness allows you to see that *you are not your addiction.* This approach also includes meditations that enhance people's positive feelings, particularly towards themselves—something we all recognize in psychology as self-acceptance or self-esteem. The mindfulness approach has been used effectively with mental illnesses like schizophrenia,[78] and it is now being applied to addiction along with mental illness.[79] Alan Marlatt's group at the University of Washington has used mindfulness to combat cravings that lead to relapse.[80]

Approaches focused on your ability to function, how you cope with the world, and your ways of thinking about yourself align perfectly with what we know about human behavior. Here research agrees with what seems logical, even irrefutable. You are enormously more likely to beat addiction if you feel strong and capable—if you embrace and nurture your own power. This is what The PERFECT Program does.

There is nothing and no one more able than you to begin and sustain your recovery

The disease model presents itself as an enlightened view of addiction that does not stigmatize or undermine the addict. But that claim is bogus. The PERFECT Program takes the opposite approach to the impossible disease model idea that you must accept that you're powerless in order to begin recovery. In order to recover, you don't need to learn to think like an addict. Instead, *you need to learn to think like a non-addict.* And your life-seeking, healthy core is the engine of your recovery.

Moving Forward

So now you know these facts: (1) thinking of yourself as an addict isn't necessary and serves only as an additional burden to overcoming your problem, (2) the best science shows that you are more likely to overcome your addiction than not, (3) the seeds for doing so are already within you—everything human about you and everything you know of life is part of what will enable you to overcome addiction. From here on, The PERFECT Program—building on the best evidence from effective treatments—will help you harness and direct your life force toward recovery.

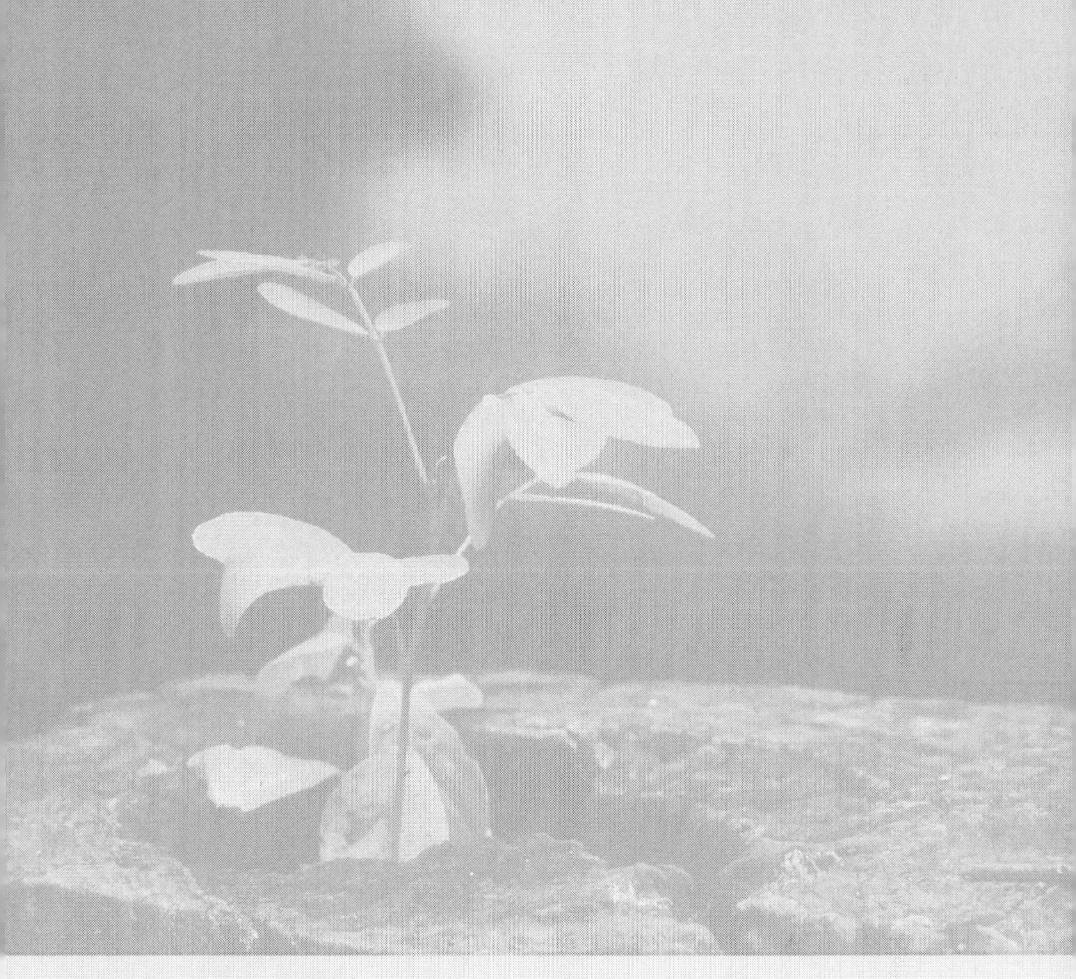

PART II
THE PERFECT PROGRAM

CHAPTER 3

Preparing for Change

Getting yourself ready for The PERFECT Program

CHAPTER GOALS

- To gather yourself, your materials, your resources for The PERFECT Program
- To assess your addiction, your values, your resources for change
- To define your terms of recovery, to consider your options, and to set your goals

Purpose: This chapter brings you to the starting point of your change effort. It gets you prepared, sharpens your pencils, and sets aside the space—emotionally and physically—to begin to change and to quit your addiction. You will start by assessing your addiction, defining recovery, and setting your goals. Once you start in this positive direction, you will begin moving forward steadily.

CASE: Alex had been getting drunk most nights for several years, stumbling home from his neighborhood bar, often not remembering doing so. Sometimes he found bruises and cuts that he had no memory of incurring. He decided—recognized—he was an addicted alcoholic. This wasn't an intellectual calculation. It was a decision to change.

Alex had heard terrible stories about detoxing—that it was horrid, even life-threatening. Beyond that, what would he do instead of drinking? But the fear of withdrawal overshadowed the latter concern in Alex's calculations—after all, if he could kick his alcohol habit, surely he'd find new things with which to fill his time!

And, so, Alex prepared himself well, at least for detoxing. He loaded his refrigerator with fruit juice and mineral water. He had on hand large quantities of fruits and cereals. The cereals, he reckoned, were the easiest things he could get down no matter how nauseous he became; the fruits, the healthiest things. And he recruited his brother, Paul, to stay with him in his spare bedroom.

The first weekend was hell on wheels, especially at night. Alex couldn't find comfortable sleep and he awoke throughout the night with nightmares. His hands shook when he tried to read. Several times he thought of getting his brother in the next room to drive him to the hospital.

But he also slept—fitfully—over several days. Alex actually didn't come out of his bedroom until Monday morning and then reluctantly, his eyes bloodshot, feeling sluggish and ill. Paul looked up and, calling him "sleeping beauty," told Alex he had looked in on him several times and found him sleeping—albeit sometimes thrashing.*

This case is simply an affirmation of truths borne out by history and science. Many, many people have quit many, many addictions before the creation of the Betty Ford Center. The most important reality for you to embrace is this: You are not your addiction. You are not *an addict.* Your true self is the engine of your recovery. The essence of The PERFECT Program is to fortify the *real you* to take the reins of your life.

---

* Caution: I am not recommending that people undergo medically unsupervised detoxification the way Alex—or Rose (meth)—did. See note 1 for a discussion of alcohol withdrawal.

Getting Ready

Materials

This chapter is going to put you to work delving into the essence of your addiction, getting you back in touch with the things that give your life value and purpose, and establishing some goals. Let's get started by clearing some space and gathering supplies. Here's what you'll need:

Two journals. One is for personal writing and one for completing the PERFECT exercises and tracking progress. We'll call them your Personal Journal and your PERFECT Journal. You can use any kind of notebook or pad, but make sure that it is something that appeals to you and is functional so that you'll be inspired to use it. Most importantly, dedicate your journals to this process and keep them free of extraneous notes like to-do lists or random phone numbers—anything that will distract your mind with unfinished tasks. You might even get a **third notebook** for jotting down tasks and items that occur to you as you are using your dedicated journals. This will allow you to clear them from your mind for the time being and put them in a safe place that you can revisit later. Similarly, choose **writing implements** that feel good to use, with free-flowing ink, and keep them with your journal so you don't have to go scrounging for pens. If you prefer, you can start a journal on your computer or start a private blog. Keep it front and center on your desktop so that it is easily accessible, or set your computer to open your journal at start-up.

A timer. This will come in handy for some of The PERFECT exercises. Don't use your alarm clock, unless you have one with a pleasing tone that won't jangle your nerves. Egg timers can be purchased for under five dollars, or you can even use the timer on your cell phone set to a gentle chime. There are also meditation timer apps for cell phones.

A meditation spot. Meditation is a central element of The PERFECT Program (don't panic—we'll walk you through it), and you'll want to create a space where you can sit without distraction.

You don't have to create a shrine or invest in an expensive silk and buckwheat cushion—unless you are inspired to do so. All you need is a quiet spot and half an hour to yourself. You can sit on a pillow on the floor, on a straight-backed chair, or even under a tree. (Now, if it's under a tree, you'll need an indoor and an outdoor spot, for when weather forbids communing with nature!) Make sure it's a spot where you can relax. For instance, if you choose a place next to the cat box or a pile where you collect dirty laundry, you won't want to spend time there.

How does addiction appear in your life?

Addiction manifests differently in everyone, and for different reasons. Addiction includes a wide range of involvements, whether with substances or behaviors, and its causes and effects are both specific and complex. Rather than tell you what your problem is and present you with one solution, we're going to guide you through the process of assessing your addiction and the impact it has on your life—remembering that it can be more or less severe. Once you are clear about where you stand, you can begin to set some goals, and PERFECT will guide you through that process, too.

Recovery does not have to look like endless days of white-knuckle abstinence and a procession of tedious meetings. If addiction is a treadmill, then recovery is a grand adventure. Understanding that addiction is a destructive, self-negating, ingrained behavior chosen in response to life circumstances and that recovery means infusing your life with a sense of purpose, personal agency, and new skills, you can create a broader vision of what your personal recovery will look like. Through The PERFECT Program, you will be creating a life for yourself that is utterly incompatible with addiction, replacing self-destructive patterns with life-affirming pursuits. Recall Rose (in Chapter 1) as an example. Despite her reverence for her child, her lifestyle allowed addiction in. She rebuilt a life around family (parents, child, and eventually husband), positive social groups (her single mothers' group), education, marriage, and a career that ruled out her addiction forever.

Let's begin by assessing your addiction and making some decisions about what freedom from addiction will mean for you. You will need your PERFECT Journal for this.

ADDICTION SELF-ASSESSMENT QUESTIONNAIRE

1. **What substance(s) or behavior(s) are you addicted to?**
   - If you have more than one, list them from the one that has the most negative and consuming impact on your life to the least.

2. **Focusing on the addiction at the top of your list:**
   - How often do you engage in your addictive behavior?
   - If you use a substance, how much do you use at a time? If it is a behavior, describe your involvement in detail. How often do you rely on it?
   - At what times of the day or under what circumstances do you do it, typically?
   - When you are not engaged in the substance or behavior of your addiction, when and how much do you think about it?
   - For how long have you had this level of involvement with your addiction?

3. **Now go through all the questions in #2 with the next most virulent addiction on your list.**

4. **What experience are you seeking through your addiction(s)? Describe your feelings when using, or when you're involved in the activity. Summarize what it does for you or gives you.**
   - Do you actually achieve this experience? If so, how often and for how long?
   - What other experiences come with your addiction? List both positive and negative.

5. **How does your addiction impact your daily life?**
   - Family and friends?
   - Responsibilities?
   - Leisure time?
   - Finances?
   - Health?
   - Self-esteem?

6. When is your addiction at its peak? What is going on in your life at those times?

7. Are there periods during which your addiction seems to be less powerful? If so, when? What is different about these times?

8. Have you ever stopped your addiction for a period? For how long? How did your stopping affect your life? How did you feel?

9. Do you believe that you can overcome your addiction? Why do you think you can or can't?

10. At this moment, imagine what it would be like living without this addictive involvement, and describe that life.

VALUES QUESTIONNAIRE

1. Name three things that are important to you, whether or not you are actively honoring them right now.

2. What activities would you be pursuing if you were not so occupied with your addiction?

3. Have you abandoned any dreams because of your addiction? If so, name these.

4. What are some things you value that you could lose in the future due to your addiction?

5. What do you hold close to your heart that most opposes your addiction (religious faith, parenthood, political activism, health, self-respect, regard for others, etc.)?

6. What key skills or talents do you have?

7. What are your most positive qualities?

8. Name at least two accomplishments or events that you are proud of: Did you help someone? Did you win a competition? Did you build or create something? Did you stand up for something you believe in?

9. Who are the most important people in your life, either people you really care about, or people you can really count on, or both?

10. Which three human values do you elevate most, such as kindness, generosity, friendship, honesty, hard work, creativity, independence, integrity?

Withdrawal

The physical journey

If you think of your body as a collection of chemicals responding to one another and working in unison, it makes sense that introducing a new chemical into the mix is going to force all the other chemicals to respond to it. Many people remember feeling disgusted by their first encounter with cigarettes—nauseous and light-headed, perhaps. That's simply the body's response to a chemical interloper disturbing the body's balance. But after continued use, the body will adjust and begin working with this new chemical in order to reestablish its equilibrium. Now, the body comes to expect this chemical and complains if it doesn't receive it. That complaint takes the form of withdrawal.

It's standard to call this situation "physical dependence" or "chemical dependence," but the word "dependence" is misleading. The body is dependent on water for survival, but could never be dependent on nicotine or alcohol for survival. "Accustomed" is a more accurate word. While it is true that some people have developed such a high tolerance for their drug of choice that withdrawal can be medically risky, less severe withdrawal is the rule.* The more likely scenario is that you will experience

---

*In these extreme cases, particularly involving hypnotic-depressants (especially alcohol and benzodiazepines), medically supervised detox is a wise option. If you have any concerns about this, please consult with a doctor who is experienced in this area, and who is not in AA himself or herself (unless they are capable of separating themselves from their personal experience). Under any circumstances notify someone close to you about your plans, and in extreme cases arrange for them to stay with you. See note 1 for a discussion of alcohol withdrawal.

some discomfort while your body adjusts. It will be unpleasant, and then it will be over. Of course, you must be immediately sensitive if this is not the case and be prepared to get medical help. In any case, it is after this phase that you will face the long-term challenge of dealing with your real life—the one beyond your addiction.

If you are giving up a drug, but not only then (see love withdrawal, below), fear of withdrawal may be a major hurdle that prevents you from pursuing recovery.[1] The fact is that withdrawal can be miserable. You might be facing a few days of physical and mental discomfort: restlessness or insomnia, headaches, shakes, digestive problems, nausea, depression, anxiety, even grief. There are things you can do to help you cope in the short run, including having someone aware of your situation who can look after you as needed, but even more importantly for the duration:

- Arrange to have positive outings and experiences, things that always bring you pleasure
- After your initial adjustment, taking perhaps a couple of days, make sure to see (certainly don't isolate yourself from) family and friends
- Arrange to see a counselor, a therapist, or a spiritual figure
- Do regular physical activity, even if minimal—like walking around the block or climbing stairs
- If cooking or engaging in formal meals seems like a stretch, nonetheless do maintain regular nutritious intake of food—think of yourself as training for a fight or race
- Remember, recall, visualize what this is all about—you're not coming off your addiction for something to do—you're heading somewhere, toward a different life, one that expresses who you really are and want to be—have those images available for ready access

"What if I'm not addicted to crack or heroin (or OxyContin), or alcohol dependent?!"

In the last section I might seem to be writing for people who have given over their lives (and all their time) to an addiction in which they've isolated themselves from civilized society. Many people who come to this book will still have jobs, families, or other daily responsibilities while facing serious addictive problems. If you are functioning in your regular roles but still anticipate disruptive withdrawal and a difficult transition and readjustment, part of your preparation will be to arrange for time off from work and/or for people to take over what you're normally expected to do, like providing meals for your kids. There is, of course, the risk of over-preparing. This is a question no one can resolve for you—including, perhaps, even you yourself. That is, anticipating great pain and discomfort that may not occur can be an unnecessary hindrance to quitting, while being unprepared for more severe withdrawal is a danger. So, always have a fallback plan in place.

CASE: Ezra was growing and wholesaling marijuana for acquaintances, mainly former co-workers he knew at the major firm where he had worked. Ezra had a family—a wife and two small children. When his kids entered preschool, he foresaw the difficulties he might have conducting his business. And, so, Ezra began the laborious process of (1) cleaning up his growing operation—the soil, the irrigation stones, the water hoses and outlets, the ruined floors beneath the tubs for the plants—what a mess! (2) cleaning himself up from his around-the-clock pot-smoking addiction.

Ezra had never slept well. Indeed, his drug use was in good part aimed at alleviating his anxiety. So he anticipated—and experienced—quite a few sleepless nights without his drug of choice. He was concerned to be rested and focused because now that he was forced once again to get a real job, he had to concentrate on creating a resume, rekindling long-lost work skills, and reconnecting with his old work network.

It was tough going for several months. But—as might be expected of someone running an urban growth operation while raising a family—Ezra was smart and resourceful. He coped. After his period of readjustment, Ezra concluded, "You know, quitting drugs wasn't all that hard." In fact, quitting gave him a chance to work on his life-long insomnia and to develop better ways to find sleep at night.

Maintain your perspective

Children come unhinged when they know they're going to get an injection at the doctor's office. They can work themselves up into such a panic over this impending apocalypse that they will scream and cry, anticipating the little pinch that hurts significantly less than a stubbed toe or a scraped knee. The actual discomfort is nothing compared to the terror that precedes it. Similarly, while you may be nervous about experiencing some physical discomfort, try to maintain your perspective on it, because your perception of that discomfort makes the difference between a tolerable and an intolerable situation. Also, remember that it's finite—it will end. You will feel better.

Care for the whole person

The point with Alex and Ezra is that, while your body is experiencing some physical symptoms, this is not the major part of the withdrawal experience. After all, people frequently quit addictions, only to relapse at some point farther down the road, when physical withdrawal is a distant memory. As Alan Marlatt showed through his research in his volume (edited with Dennis Donovan), *Relapse Prevention* (Guilford, 2005), relapse occurring after immediate withdrawal has passed is the rule.

CASE: Savannah had been addicted to heroin since her early twenties. Now in her forties, she—and those who knew her—figured quitting the drug was impossible. Sal, a friend of many years who had always known Savannah to be addicted, was one of those who believed this to be true. As almost a chance question, he asked Savannah, "Have you ever been off narcotics?" "Yeah," Savannah answered casually, "I once quit for two years." Sal had two thoughts: "She could quit!" and "Why did she go back, since it is such a misery for her to be addicted?"

As another example, peak cigarette withdrawal lasts several days, and even residual withdrawal effects not more than a month.[2] So if you relapse, it's rarely in response to bodily readjustment due to withdrawal. Relapse is caused by psychological and life issues that both exacerbate your withdrawal and persist long after it.[3]

Ezra, for example, had to cope with a quick temper that now surfaced when he had to deal with trivial issues created hourly when managing young kids—anger that marijuana had warded off for him. As it does for many people, the din of an active addiction had drowned out the painful negative commentary that loops through one's mind. These are stories you tell yourself about how strange, hopeless, or worthless you are, and they can become especially loud and insistent during this period. You might, for instance, begin berating yourself for having been addicted or insisting to yourself that it's too late for you. You might feel overwhelmed by the road ahead. It's not possible to stop these thoughts from intruding, but you can diffuse their power by recognizing them when they appear and calling them what they are. For instance, "Oh, there's that old voice telling me that I won't succeed," or "My mind is running off again." Just be aware that it happens to us all.

"How did I used to spend all my time?"

In the last chapter, I spoke of the centrality of addictions for filling and structuring one's life:

> Days planned around purchasing and consuming the substance or practicing the activity; fielding negative fallout (like angry co-workers, family members, and friends; mounting bills; health problems); making solemn promises to stop; remorse and guilt. . . . Yet, as painful and self-defeating as these feelings are, their predictability sustains addicts and even lends a bizarre sense of purpose to their lives. Rather than being a medical mystery, *addiction makes complete psychological sense.*

To say the least, people who are giving up their addictions often find themselves with a lot of time on their hands. You don't realize how all-consuming an addiction is—how much time it devours—until you're sitting there with the whole day and night stretched out in front of you, and the next fifteen minutes seem like an eternity. This is the time to indulge in some simple pleasures. Rent some movies; stock up on engrossing novels; make plans to meet with friends for coffee or breakfast; embark on a project you've been meaning to tackle, like learning to play the ukulele, starting a garden, or painting the bathroom. Plan your day and create as much structure as possible.

But, in addition, you are going to have to create—or re-create—a non-addicted life structure based on a larger vision of yourself. And you will have plenty of time now to concentrate on that task, which you and I will work on in the following sections of this book.

Seek support

The Substance Abuse and Mental Health Services Administration (SAMHSA, the agency responsible for the National Survey on Drug Use and Health referred to in the previous chapter) has recently redefined recovery. In 2011, the agency reversed decades of thinking to create a "new working definition of recovery from mental and substance use disorders":

> Recovery is a process of change whereby individuals work to improve their own health and wellness and to live a meaningful life in a community of their choice while striving to achieve their full potential.[4]

SAMHSA's redefinition creates "four pillars of recovery: health, home, purpose, and community."[5] "Purpose" means that recovery is self-activated—including finding "meaningful daily activities, such as a job, school, volunteerism, family caretaking, or creative endeavors, and the independence, income and resources to participate in society."

Community and support constitute one of the essential pillars of recovery. This is the time to begin building (and rebuilding) your personal community. In Britain (more so than in the United States—go figure) a therapy measured to be as effective as the motivational enhancement that I discussed in the last chapter is called "social network therapy" (also social behavior and network therapy). This therapy involves finding or creating a supportive, non-addictive community and social contacts.[6] During the immediate quitting period, you can turn to supportive family and friends; let them know how they can help. Remember Rose's mom and Alex's brother. Then there is involvement in larger communities, like Ezra reemerging into the work world, or your helping others, joining a church, finding a support group (like Rose's single mothers' group), a hiking club, and on and on. This pillar dovetails with finding meaningful activities—including work, school, volunteering, family caretaking, creative endeavors—that provide you with the independence and resources to participate in society.

People Don't Really Withdraw from Love (Do They?)

I was teaching at the Harvard Business School while writing *Love and Addiction* before its publication in 1975. One of my colleagues there, who had seen an interview I had done in the *Boston Globe*, walked by me and laughed, "Right, love addiction!" Yes, people become transfixed in their love affairs, sacrificing everything for them, sometimes murdering or committing suicide or tolerating ongoing abuse for the sake of what they view as a love relationship. But their chagrin, pain, and dissociation often reach highest pitch when a love affair ends. One of my most popular posts at *Psychology Today Blogs* was "The 7 Hardest Addictions to Quit: Love Is the Worst!"[7] Yes, that's right—worse than heroin, cocaine, or smoking. Without repeating the arguments in my blogpost, let me reprint a comment from a reader:

> My divorce has left me completely blindsided and affected every aspect of my life. It is something that I have struggled for years to get over and to this day cannot seem to move forward. It has literally destroyed so much of me and continues to take another piece day by day. I fear what the outcome will be in the end.

Or, from the *New York Times*:

> In 12-step confessional style, this is what love addiction did to my life: I dropped out of college, quit my job, stopped talking to my family and friends. There was no booze to blame for my blackouts, vomiting and bed-wetting. No pills to explain the 15 hours a day I slept. No needles as excuse for my alarming weight loss. I hit bottom one sleepless night, strung out on the bedroom floor, contemplating suicide. And then I spent four months—and a good chunk of my family's money—in treatment for love addiction.[8]

And on and on. I know my colleague at Harvard would probably sneer at these. Or else you might say, "Well, these people have preexisting psychiatric conditions." Yes, more or less like many other addicts. To state it briefly, people become addicted to an entire gestalt of feelings, physical reactions, and experiences. No one element can be separated from any other. Emergence from that gestalt may be earth-shattering. As I wrote in *The Meaning of Addiction*:

> Neither traumatic drug withdrawal nor a person's craving for a drug is exclusively determined by physiology. Rather, the experience both of a felt need (or craving) for and of withdrawal from an object or involvement engages a person's expectations, values, and self-concept, as well as the person's sense of alternative opportunities for gratification. These complications are introduced not out of disillusionment with the notion of addiction but out of respect for its potential power and utility. Suitably broadened and strengthened, the concept of addiction provides a powerful description of human behavior, one that opens up important opportunities for understanding not only drug abuse, but compulsive and self-destructive behaviors of all kinds.[9]

Choosing Your Goals

For generations now, it's been gospel that overcoming addiction requires resigning yourself to abstaining, come hell or high water. Yet, at the same time, recovery is often punctuated with dangerous binge relapses like Amy Winehouse's. This whole sequence occurs because conventional recovery means making your addiction continue to be the absolute center of your universe by the continual, perpetual rejection or negation of it—like the anorexic who used to be overweight. Life was about being addicted, and now it's about fighting being addicted, which often resembles being addicted, as some people note about the way many alcoholics use AA.

Either way, the addiction is the core around which your whole life revolves. It's a grim picture, so it's no wonder so many people reject it. Even if your ultimate goal is complete abstinence—which it may be, considering the nature of your addiction and your priorities in life—there are more effective, empowering, and life-affirming ways of achieving it. Once you realize that addiction is not about the power that a substance or compulsion has over you, a horizon of possibilities for recovery opens up.

Self-control and free will

Recover! is not a discussion of free will—after all, I'm a psychologist, not a philosopher! It's about the skills and outlooks you need to recover. But the recovery field has a special angle on free will—they use a term in AA called "self-will," which they see as a negative. Contrary to this finger-wagging disempowerment, true recovery from addiction means reclaiming your power and free will, not giving it up. Exercising free will is not just doing what you feel like doing or acting on every whim or craving or desire. Rather, it means making choices and pursuing actions based on your values and priorities, *in spite of whims and feelings to the contrary.* Twelve-step recovery says you can't do this; I know and you know that you can. Imagine that it's the day before you're scheduled to take a certification exam. If you pass, you will qualify for a dream job that will allow you to provide for your family. You have to study and go to bed early, but you're burned out and really feel like watching all the episodes of your favorite series on CD or the Internet. Choosing to turn off the video and study is a true act of self-will, while planting yourself on the couch with a bucket of hot wings is, in this case, an abdication of will.

You can watch your series and eat hot wings another time. Delay of gratification, it's called. Its absence is central to addiction, and being able to delay gratification is often crucial for recovery. For addiction means giving in to the appeal of a simple solution, the addictive experience, whenever confronted with difficult emotions or life issues, rather than seeking out harder, long-term (real) solutions for these things. Remember, Rose couldn't confront her long-term issues and goals, and so she used meth instead. Impulsiveness—yet another term for the tendency just to reach for a reward or experience—has often been seen as playing a role in addiction. Remember our discussion in Chapter 2 of impulsiveness, the brain's frontal lobes, and the addicted and non-addicted siblings and their dysfunctional inferior frontal gyrus. Impulsiveness and its opposite are more than the equipment you are born with.

People often learn—or don't learn—the ability to delay gratification early in life, as children. Cultural commentators have become very concerned that American children—compared with those in France, for example[10]—don't learn how to delay gratification. This may be connected to the obesity epidemic in this country, among other things. Another term for this is self-control, which is kind of the down-to-earth, day-to-day version of free will. This exercise of free will takes effort. But, here's the great thing—modern cognitive science shows that self-control improves with practice, and best sellers are now being written explaining this.[11] Self-control and delay of gratification can certainly be instilled in children.[12]

As with everything else associated with addiction—indeed, with life—meaning is crucial. It is when people feel that self-control is valuable and fulfilling that—although it may require sacrifice at a given moment—they are more willing to exercise it. Think about requiring children to dust and vacuum as chores. It works better to make them responsible for keeping an area clean and organized when completing a project or because the area is a place where they play or carry out activities. When cleaning and being responsible for an area (or the entire house) connects to their own desires and goals, the task *has meaning for them*—it is really no longer a task. Similarly, as you work your way into your non-addicted life and begin to savor its effects and benefits in areas that you enjoy and seek to improve, your motivation is reinforced and expands—that is the recovery pillar called purpose.

I am taking pains to make these points and to draw this distinction because the disease theory has made "willpower" a dirty word. Trying to develop and to rely on your own willpower seems to go against the scientific notion of the hijacked brain that we considered in Chapter 2, or the rejection of "self-will" by the 12-step movement. After all, relying on your own will violates the third Step: "Made a decision to turn our will and our lives over to the care of God as we understood Him." This three-card-monte switcheroo—calling the exercise of free will a cause of rather than a remedy for addiction—undermines success in overcoming addiction by leading people to believe that, as diseased addicts, their spirit is broken and self-direction is a path leading them back to addiction.

In fact, true recovery means shifting the balance of power *away* from addiction and toward your own free will. Taking the focus off the substance or behavior and putting it back where it belongs—on your values and sense of life purpose—allows you to determine what recovery means for you. Keep in mind that the opposite of addiction is not abstinence. The opposite of addiction is intention and what you seek in your life, and there is nothing wrong with your ability to determine these things for yourself and to pursue them. Your recovery goals should represent who you are and what's meaningful to you, although you can always revisit and change your goals as you progress down this path. The PERFECT Program makes clear that your recovery is your own creation. This kind of true recovery is going to look different for every person. I use the term "recovery" because it's a familiar term—but remember that it's also a loaded word. In fact, it might be helpful to replace it in your mind with ideas like *balance* or *self-direction*, and to imagine this as a process of displacing addiction with things you want that you know will improve your life.

CASE: Let's go back to the new, detoxed Alex—the one who went through scary alcohol withdrawal but emerged to see his brother at the breakfast table, and then faced the rest of his life (he was thirty-two). Now what?

Along with a family (including his parents, brother, and sister), Alex had a girlfriend, Susan. He also had a job, at which he continued, only now without facing hangovers in the mornings. Susan wasn't an alcoholic, but went out many evenings with Alex, drinking far less by his side. She was younger (twenty-three), and perhaps that explained her acceptance of Alex's extreme drinking. In any case—and thankfully for Alex—it didn't put her off the relationship. So, when Alex told her he was quitting drinking, Susan wondered, "How will we spend our evenings now?"

In fact, Alex relied on Susan for much of the answer to that question. She had her own family, circle of friends, and things she did with both—and on her own—like going to movies, staying home and sewing, and going to the gym. Alex turned to Susan as if he was seeking a navigator through foreign territory for guidance as to what people who don't spend their nights drinking do. And she now took Alex under her wing, as much as was reasonable (he didn't begin sewing, although he did start reading while Susan sewed).

Abstinence

In regards to your addiction itself, what are you shooting for? Never to use again—complete, lifelong abstinence—is one goal. It is a quite difficult goal to achieve, but it may perhaps be advisable, depending upon what you're addicted to, the state of your psychological and physical health, and what is most important to you. Still, it's important to keep in mind that abstinence means *not* doing something. Abstinence has no inherent value except as it aligns with what's valuable or meaningful for you to pursue. In other words, recovery is not a purity test, and abstinence is not the holy grail. It's important to make this distinction because recovery culture has an abstinence fetish, a belief that in order to be considered "sober" people must be free of all mind-altering substances, renewing their commitment to abstinence on a daily basis for the rest of their lives. And yes, this includes people in their teens or early twenties.

Let's look at the word "sobriety." In the real world, sobriety means not being impaired. In 12-step speak, sobriety means never taking any consciousness-altering substance, *ever*. This fixation on abstinence requires that people who recover through the 12 steps decide that their lives revolve around an empty space. Not only is that undesirable, it's unsustainable. You can't commit your life to nothingness, only to health, your goals and plans, and your belief in yourself.

As a marker of other progress rather than an essential goal in itself, abstinence is not a state of grace. If you're striving for abstinence but you go off the wagon, you have not blown your recovery or ruined everything; you do not have to "start over." There is no such thing as starting over. This is your life we're talking about, not a contest. Here's an analogy: Imagine your whole life spread out in front of you like a sea of clear water. Now, imagine that you pour a bottle of red wine in. The wine will diffuse fairly rapidly and disappear into the vastness of the sea, and the impact will be absorbed. Now imagine that you have narrowed the scope to one day, represented by a single pail of water. When you pour a bottle of wine in, the water is unable to diffuse it. This is the difference between true recovery and living an endless string of one-day-at-a-time reprieves.

CASE: Alex decided to spend a night drinking again after more than six months of abstinence. He wanted to see what it felt like. Susan prepared to accompany him for the evening. And so, dressed for battle, the two went to Alex's favorite pub. For one thing, Alex didn't have to pay for a drink. All his old drinking cronies stopped by their table and ordered one for him.

But, truth be told, Alex was finding it hard to consume so many drinks. First, he didn't order anything for Susan, but passed the extras along to her. Alex ended up having five drinks, and Susan three. And it was only 9:30! Looking around ruefully, Alex indicated to Susan that it was time to go. With terse farewells to his former fellow revelers, Alex and Susan went out the door of the bar. "Is it too late to catch a movie?" Alex asked Susan.

If you choose abstinence for yourself, make it an empowered choice, unencumbered by the neurotic trappings of conventional recovery. Choose abstinence, not because it is the only way for all addicts, but because:

- It is genuinely what you desire.
- You violate your values using, in the presence of, or in pursuit of the behavior or substance.
- The behavior or substance is genuinely dangerous to you or others.
- The substance is illegal or life disrupting in other ways.
- Moderate involvement is not a realistic possibility for you.

Most important to keep in mind is that abstinence serves your life plan, not vice versa. This means (1) a simple violation does not indicate that you have swerved from your plan, which you can resume instantly and completely; (2) you can revise your plan. In Alex's case, he continued to abstain, with the idea that once every six months he would go out drinking again. He did this for several years, although he never consumed on *any* of these nights anything like the amount he used to drink regularly. Years later, he decided to quit drinking altogether. Do any real alcoholics you know follow this path? Plenty; and here's one who admitted it—Christine Quinn. In a revelatory memoir she released in preparation for running for mayor of New York City, Quinn described her bulimia and drinking problem: "By the time Ms. Quinn left college . . . bingeing and purging and drinking to get drunk were regular habits."

Quinn entered and successfully completed rehab for bulimia in 1992:

> For the first time, Ms. Quinn also examined her drinking. She arrived back in New York with a meal plan and a referral to a therapist who specialized in eating disorders and alcoholism. She cut back to drinking moderately, having only the occasional glass of wine, which she continued until about three years ago [i.e., the better part of a decade], when she stopped entirely. She says she considers herself an alcoholic.[13]

Here's a more troubling example, one that I listened to at a meeting of a recovery group devoted to abstinence.

> **CASE:** Renee had been abstinent for six years. One night, leaving her supermarket parking lot, she noticed in the corner of the lot a bar that she knew had a fireplace. Since it was near Christmas, and her own apartment (which she shared with her husband) had no fireplace, she decided to drop in the bar. She had too much to drink, drove home, and was quickly stopped by the police, lost her license, and was unable to continue at her job—which led to a divorce from her husband.

This horrifying story didn't have to occur, as we will see in the relapse prevention section of The PERFECT Program. However, even taken at its worst, Renee drank too much one night in six years. She had a lot to make up for, but she didn't drink again for another four years. Getting drunk one night in a decade is about as good a record as anyone could hope for (recall the analogy of spilling a bottle of wine in the ocean). This story is not meant to make light of Renee's suffering and guilt. It is meant to put in perspective what a violation of an abstinence vow should actually mean and how it should be handled.

Moderation

It's important to understand that addiction is a coping mechanism—a destructive (but efficient) one that produces negative consequences in your life. Considering it in this way puts the emphasis where it belongs—on *you*. You are the locus of addiction, not a substance, a disease, or an outside force. For a little perspective, think of all the possible substances and behaviors people can become addicted to: powerful, mind-altering drugs; milder, mood-altering drugs; dangerous or risky behaviors; recreational activities (like gambling); everyday, even life-sustaining behaviors (like eating and sex). These things are so diverse that the only element they all share—besides sometimes being addictive—is the human one. People are resourceful enough to make just about anything the object of their addiction. In other words, whatever you're addicted to is incidental to the condition of being addicted. Being addicted is like being malnourished or depressed—it's a state you are in—a condition unto itself, while your drug or behavior is just a symptom of addiction.

This is a crucial distinction because popular addiction mythology places all the emphasis on the drug or behavior itself, insisting that addicts admit their powerlessness over the thing to which they are addicted. This mythology is focused on, instead of eliminating addiction, eliminating the symptoms or the random objects of people's addictions. From this backwards perspective, lifelong abstinence is the only option, and moderation is a crazy delusion. Consider this, however: if you are no longer addicted, and you have healthy coping strategies, there is no drug that can render you helpless before it. When addiction ends, so does the compulsion to escape. The objects of your addiction remain neutral—they are, and always have been, just things, behaviors, objects. They had no innate power before addiction, and certainly have none after. *Moderation is indeed possible for people who have truly recovered from addiction. You may be able to look forward to drinking a glass of wine or having a beer after work or eating a piece of chocolate cake or going to Las Vegas with your friends without fear of ruining your life.*

One reason we often don't hear about people who moderate their drinking is that it happens so matter-of-factly. People usually don't make a big deal of it; it's just part of the natural evolution of their lives—remember that "more than half of those [alcoholics] who have fully recovered drink at low-risk levels," as discussed in the previous chapter. As a result, this common phenomenon typically takes place under the radar, occasionally popping up in a story about a celebrity. I described how New York politician Christine Quinn cut back to drinking only an occasional glass of wine, a practice she maintained for years. Less than two weeks after Quinn's story appeared in the *New York Times*, the paper ran an interview with Billy Joel, once well known for his heavy consumption of vodka and scotch. Explaining that he doesn't "subscribe to A.A. . . . to 12-step stuff," Joel reported that currently "I have a glass of wine with a meal."[14] These two stories, appearing within a couple of weeks of each other, stand for others—many, many others.

One disproof of the "frontal lobe" theory from the previous chapter—in which Dr. Drew claims that if addicted your "brain frontality" dies or becomes comatose—is that then your brain couldn't control *any* potentially addictive activity. Really? Thus, in his podcast with harm-reduction specialists Drs. Jaffe and Kern (harm reduction is discussed in the next section), when Dr. Jaffe said that he had had a major meth habit but now drank moderately, as well as perhaps smoking marijuana, Dr. Drew was driven to make up the Jewish exception—claiming that only Ashkenazi Jews had the special genetic immunity that allowed Jaffe's feat. For the record, I know a number of non-Jewish former speed freaks who currently drink moderately—including Rose. Apparently, methamphetamines are one thing, white wine and marijuana others. In any case, it's interesting to hear Dr. Jaffe describe the anxiety with which he had a glass of champagne after he had been in treatment for his addiction and thought he had to quit every kind of psychoactive substance.[15] Many clients and others have described this apprehension to me.

Of course, aiming for moderation requires self-knowledge. For instance, for some people, there is no point to moderation. There's little value in moderation for someone whose only reason for drinking is just to get drunk. Why bother? However, someone who drinks addictively sometimes, but who also has the capacity to enjoy wine with dinner or with friends, has a good reason to see moderation as a recovery goal. It contributes value to his life. Other objects of addiction may have no value in themselves. In these cases, an activity may be readily given up in its entirety—like gambling. But it's not for me or anyone else to make that decision for you.

CASE: Tristan was a lifelong addicted gambler. His father had been one, and as a teenager he ran away to escape his dysfunctional home, but then started gambling himself. He progressed in his habit over decades until he married and had a young daughter. In his efforts to protect his family from his addiction—in what could be termed a harm-reduction step—Tristan turned his paychecks over to his wife, who allotted him an allowance. Still, a couple of nights a month, he spent all night on the

Internet gambling, sometimes throwing away thousands of dollars that he and his wife planned to use to buy a home.

Previously, Tristan would quit, then edge back into gambling, perhaps lured by an online offer or ads he saw for a casino or racetrack. When he turned forty, he despaired about ever having some of the things that eluded him and his family. In addition, he was starting his own business. Tristan went to a non-12-step therapist who didn't demand that he stop gambling. During his therapy, Tristan went on several gambling binges. Finally, he told his therapist, "I know this isn't a disease. But, whatever it is, I don't think I can control this thing. Maybe not now, or maybe ever. I need to quit." His therapist responded, "Good idea. What do you think it will take for you to stop gambling entirely? Let's describe that lifestyle, its restrictions, and replacement activities. Let's make a plan."

Two obvious points about Tristan's case are: (1) the power and meaning of his decision to abstain came from his arriving at the decision for himself, (2) his abstinence (like his urge to be addiction-free) came in the service of larger, more important goals in his life: family, career, and home.

But Tristan could give up gambling—it wasn't essential for his life. Some addicts *must* moderate, because the object of their addiction is something they cannot quit, like food, sex, or shopping. Yet, 12-step recovery has applied its short-sighted, ineffective temperance mentality to this arena of addiction, too. It does so by saying, for instance, "You must abstain from *non-marital* sex," or that one must avoid sugar, alone, of all foods. But an addiction to binge-eating cannot be cured by repeating the mantra that food is just fuel and should never be enjoyed, and that you can never have a dessert again. That's a recipe for relapse.

As to "illicit" (nonmarital) sex (including masturbation), isn't that a bit old-fashioned? What if you aren't married, or don't have a stable partner? Will you never be allowed to have sex, or an orgasm, again, like a monk or a nun? Nor can a sex addiction be cured by scheduling and micromanaging sexual encounters. That's like curing food addiction with an eating disorder, or trying not to think of the proverbial pink elephant—all of which simply sets you up for failure somewhere down the road. The goal of The PERFECT Program is to restore quality of life, which means being able to enjoy food, sex, and necessary life experiences and pleasures in a carefree manner, as you were meant to. This will happen when you restore balance and meaning to your life and learn to live with intention.

In contemplating moderation, here are some questions for you to consider:

- Is moderation a realistic option for you?
- Are you addicted to something that will contribute to your quality of life if used moderately?
- Would even moderate use jeopardize your or anyone else's safety or well-being?
- Would moderate use be more trouble than it's worth?
- What would moderation look like for you?

Abstinence and moderation (or harm reduction, as we shall see in the next section) are not distinct options, and you do not have to choose one now and forever. They are very fluid approaches to pursue in your PERFECT Program; they overlap and support each other and evolve (think of Alex and Tristan). Understanding these approaches might also give you even more clarity and insight into the nature of addiction. You might, for instance, want to be able to drink alcohol normally, but don't feel confident that moderation is possible for you right now. So, you choose to quit drinking totally for the time being while working through The PERFECT Program. When you feel ready to reintroduce alcohol, you move cautiously by instituting some brakes. Or, perhaps, you are conflicted—desiring abstinence, but afraid that you will be unable to give up your addiction. You might continue drinking but institute harm reduction safeguards, including drinking only in safe environments or under supervision and setting goals for yourself along the way.

There are infinite variations and possibilities. Addiction manifests differently in different people, and so does recovery. Taking what you have learned so far about the nature of addiction, the depth of your involvement, and the elements of your life that are most valuable, you need to set your goals—which we'll see to at the end of the chapter. I'll guide you through this process, but since recovery is not a one-size-fits-all endeavor, it is up to you to decide what approach is most appropriate for you. Remember, nothing you decide here is set in stone. You can always reassess your goals, which Dr. Jaffe did when he started drinking moderately after quitting meth; we will now examine other examples of this.

Harm reduction

Harm reduction is a policy favored by leading experts in the addiction field. It means minimizing the damage done by addiction—or any substance use—and preventing its worst potential outcomes.[16] People recover from bad nights, even bad patches and years. Some things they don't recover from. These worst outcomes—like death, AIDS, accidents, and injuries—must be avoided above all. As one example, many teens get drunk. We don't like this phenomenon, but nearly all these kids will recover (as you and I did)—unless they have an accident. Preventing accidents by avoiding drunk driving—for example, by having an arrangement that your child should call you if they have been drinking—is harm reduction. Another example of harm reduction—one more common for college students—is to have another person nearby if someone goes to sleep extremely drunk.

CASE: Ryan was talking. "Sybil was the most obnoxious girl in our crowd at college. I couldn't stand her! She never stopped talking, and what she said really never made sense. But, one night, I got drunker than I ever had. Sybil took me home, put me to bed, and slept on the sofa in my room. In the middle of the night, I was on my back, and I vomited. Sybil jumped up, made me get up out of my stupor, cleaned me up, and made me wash out my mouth and drink some water. Then we both went back to sleep. The next morning, we went out for breakfast—on me. Later one of my friends who saw us said, 'Did you sleep with Sybil? I never thought I'd see the day!' I said, 'Oh, Sybil's okay.' And I thought, 'She's more than okay—she saved my life.'"

And, so, you should—and might want to—quit your alcoholism or addiction, or abstain from alcohol or another addictive substance or activity altogether. But you can't or you won't do so now. In the meantime, you must take care of yourself. For most people, drinking or using at home is safer than going out and getting intoxicated, certainly when you are in unfamiliar territory or driving. Another risk factor is using the amount (of alcohol, narcotics) to which you were formerly accustomed after a forced period of abstinence in treatment or prison. This behavior is actually encouraged by the "in for a dime, in for a dollar" message that one drink is as bad as—the equivalent of—an all-night bender. Different substances carry with them a variety of risks in different situations—overdose, accidents, violence, withdrawal, illness, and communicable diseases—against which you must exercise care and vigilance.[17]

The key example of harm reduction in the drug field is the provision of clean needles to addicts, which reined in the spread of HIV and hepatitis among intravenous drug users and those who come into contact with them in countries—virtually every Western nation—that adopted such programs. Despite the evident common sense of harm reduction efforts, black-and-white thinking has stymied its introduction into public policy in the United States. And, so, after the initial wave of the AIDS epidemic among gay men, America became the leading economically advanced nation in numbers of new HIV cases, especially pediatric AIDS cases spread from parents to children, as the epidemic moved from homosexual men to IV drug users, often in inner cities. Tragically, this has led—and continues to lead—to thousands of unnecessary deaths. The tragedy is exacerbated because research has shown that, not only does the provision of clean needles prevent HIV from spreading, it also brings many addicts into contact with health care providers through whom they then progress to quitting their addiction altogether.[18]

Although America's abstinence fixation and perfectionism prevent us as a nation from implementing harm reduction wholeheartedly for narcotic addicts, no one is stopping you from implementing harm reduction techniques in your own life. So you must take steps to stop things from getting worse due to your addiction and to prevent incurring any permanent damage. This may mean cutting back and taking other safety precautions, even when your best goal might be to quit altogether. I don't want you, like Amy Winehouse, who died drinking heavily after leaving rehab, to kill yourself for an unachievable (for now) ideal.[19]

CASE: Lorraine was a raging alcoholic for many years. At her worst, she went on binges, disappearing overnight, where none of her family knew where she was. Her husband took to hiding the keys to her car. She thought about suicide. When friends suggested AA, she spat out a "no." Those closest to her thought she was a goner, another casualty of alcoholism.

That didn't happen to Lorraine. For a combination of reasons—family support, a job she liked, just plain self-regard (or self-will)—she bottomed out without hitting bottom, and pirouetted gradually upwards. As one key example, although she had regularly lost jobs over the years, now she enrolled in an ambitious professional graduate school program—and passed her first two years with flying colors!

But Lorraine didn't desist from drinking, or even from periodically overdrinking. What she *did* do was cut out the stupid drunk episodes. She didn't drive, or leave the house, when drunk. Instead, when she had too much to drink, she called her closest friend, Ellen.

At first Ellen was really troubled by these calls, thinking, "Am I enabling her to continue drinking, and to be an alcoholic? I was concerned for a while that she was *never* going to get better, except that she *did* get better."

By chance, Ellen read about harm reduction and so learned there was such a thing as reducing really dangerous drinking and its life-threatening consequences. Only then could she relax and help a friend whom she loved, and who continued to improve.

Among the myths of addiction is that alcoholics and other addicts can't control their consumption once they have begun drinking and using. Study after study has shown this to be false, that not only will alcoholics and others control themselves in specific circumstances, but that—when they instead consume to the point of intense intoxication—this was not an unintended consequence but their plan from the get-go.[20] Think, for example, of rules that require people to go outside their work sites in order to smoke. Objections were raised that people couldn't limit and control their addiction that way throughout the workday, given the tension that accompanies many jobs. In fact, virtually en masse, even the most committed smokers have adapted to this requirement. We (you and I) will make use of this collection of facts and information when we plan your triage and relapse prevention techniques farther along in your PERFECT Process.

There is a larger myth: that anything but abstinence is evidence of denial or self-delusion and that you really can't make any headway in fighting your addiction or improving your life without instantly quitting forever. This purity fetishism has prevented many addicted people from making the positive changes in their lives they *are* capable of (as Lorraine did), and has prevented friends and family (like Ellen) from helping them make changes that might save their lives or the lives of others or get them started in the direction of complete recovery. No matter what your ultimate goal, or whether you feel ready to leave your addiction behind, you can begin making improvements in your life immediately.

Harm Reduction Exercise

Have a look at your Addiction Self-Assessment Questionnaire, and review your answers to question 5, "How does addiction impact your daily life?" While you read your answers, ask yourself if there are changes you can make right now that will minimize the impact your behavior is having in any of these areas. A change might mean altering a pattern—for instance, choosing to smoke outside, away from family members or pets—or it might mean incorporating something new into your life, like a daily walk. Start by focusing on changing one thing. For example, you don't have to stop drinking to stop driving drunk.

Make a list of doable changes you can implement immediately that will orient you in the direction of your goals

Decide which changes you'd like to make right away and begin. It takes time for new habits to stick, so don't consider yourself a failure if you're not consistent right away. Just keep correcting, as you do with your car's steering wheel. Use your PERFECT Journal to track your progress.

GOALS WORKSHEET

1. Long-Term Goals

a. Visualize your ideal life and write about it in as much detail as possible. You might describe what a typical day of freedom looks like, for example.

2. Short-Term Goals

b. On one line, name three areas of your life that are suffering because of your addiction and, under each one, list some possible changes you can make right now to spark improvement in those areas.

c. Read over your options—some of them will be ambitious and some will be practical. Choose the one change from each list that seems most doable to you. For instance, if you are sedentary and concerned about your health, choosing to train for a 5K might sound inspiring, but a more realistic goal might be to start walking three times a week.

d. Now, under each of your choices, make note of things that will help you achieve these goals. To continue with the example above, what would you need to begin walking? A pair of sturdy but comfortable shoes? Some motivating music queued up on your MP3 player? A walking schedule? A walking buddy? A dog (you can always borrow a neighbor's, and your neighbor will thank you)? Begin gathering your resources.

e. Set a day to start implementing each of these changes, and set up a tracking system. You can use a calendar, a daily checklist, or your PERFECT Journal. There are even websites out there (like http://www.43things.com) that help you set goals, track your progress, and connect with others who share your goals. A free online calendar, like Google or Yahoo, will allow you to send reminders to yourself.

f. Remember that making these changes points you in the direction of true recovery. You are aligning yourself with your values. If you miss a day or slack off, just pick the ball back up. Every moment is an opportunity to make a positive choice.

3. Mid-Range Goals

g. Consider the journal entry you wrote on your vision for yourself, and make a list of goals you will need to meet to actualize your vision. For example, if you see yourself earning a degree, you will need to begin researching programs and requirements. Do you have to earn your GED or take the GRE?

h. Are there things you can do right now to begin preparing? If not, when would be a realistic time to begin? Write down that date.

4. Addiction Goals

Taking all your answers into consideration, what is your ultimate goal in regard to the actual substance or behavior you are addicted to? What is the best way for you to achieve that? For instance, if you are aiming for abstinence, is it more realistic *for you* to taper off, implement harm reduction methods, or go cold turkey? If you are aiming for moderation, is that a long-term goal? If so, how will you handle your addiction in the meantime? Compose a plan for yourself now, listing your addiction goals and the avenue you want to take there. Remember, you can always go back and revise as you gain clarity about yourself and your values. You are not doomed by your biological destiny—or anything else—to remain the same person you are now forever.

CASE: The rabble-rousing Irish actor, Richard Harris, came within an inch of snuffing out his life due to his cocaine addiction and alcoholism after he achieved early stardom in the 1970s. By the late 1980s, although he had survived his addictions, Harris's career had not been so fortunate, and he hadn't made a movie in years. But Harris began a concerted effort to be cast in the 1990 film *The Field*, for which he received an Academy Award nomination, and his career was rekindled, including parts in *Unforgiven*, *Gladiator*, and, most notably, the role of Albus Dumbledore in the first two Harry Potter movies.

Having made it by this time to his seventies, Harris had calmed down considerably. In an interview for *People*, Harris described resuming drinking late in life. First he described how the Dumbledore part had made him a hero to his grandchildren. And, then, he told about having a Guinness at the local pub every now and again, saying his relatives wouldn't believe it knowing he was above ground and wasn't enjoying the national beverage. Think he would blow it at this point and ruin his grandfatherly image? Apparently, that wasn't a possibility. And, so, Richard Harris died non-abstinently, but without resuming his addiction to substances.

Being human means that you are a creature in flux, that you always have the potential for change, when you are in the right place and when your personal signs tell you.

Moving Forward

You did a lot of challenging work in this chapter, exploring your life from several different angles and delving deeply into areas that might not have seen the light of day in a while. This is an enormous accomplishment, and you should take a moment now to congratulate yourself. You have compiled a valuable store of information. At this point, you should have:

- A realistic assessment of your addiction
- An understanding of how addiction impacts your life
- A (re)collection of the things that bring meaning and value to your life
- A vision of your life, free from addiction, that aligns with your values
- Short- and long-term benchmarks, guiding you toward your vision

Remember that your trajectory will be fluid. You might take a few missteps or reevaluate your goals, so it's important to broaden your scope to see that—in the big picture—your momentum is forward. In the next chapter, you will begin building the foundation of your PERFECT Program by rediscovering and fortifying your core self to take charge of your life.

LET'S GO!

CHAPTER 4

Pause

Mindfulness—Learning to listen to yourself

CHAPTER GOALS

- To learn to distinguish between addictive and healthy urges
- To recognize options and crossroads
- To activate your free will
- To begin a practice of mindfulness meditation

Purpose: This chapter helps you develop the skill of mindfulness, which means paying attention to the world and to yourself, including your addictive urges, so that you can create the space in which to recognize your addictive cravings, reconsider your options, and make life-affirming choices.

CASE: Ozzie had smoked four packs of unfiltered cigarettes a day ever since he was eighteen. Now forty-two, he had inhaled quite a bit of nicotine as he fixed televisions over that quarter century: "My hands were a filthy yellow I could never wash out," he said. Ozzie was a union activist, a shop steward, so that it was his job to stand up for fellow workers when any got in trouble. Ozzie believed in the labor movement and resolutely defended the rights of the working man against corporations. In retaliation for these efforts, Ozzie believed, the local management of the large corporation that employed him sent him to the worst parts of the city to repair TVs.

One day, while having lunch with a group of fellow workers, Ozzie went as usual to a machine to buy cigarettes. It was the early 1960s, and the price of a pack had just risen from $.30 to $.35, which one of Ozzie's fellow employees kibitzed: "They could raise the price to a dollar, and Ozzie would still pay it. The tobacco companies have Ozzie by the ________." Ozzie responded, "You're right. After this pack, I'll never buy another cigarette or smoke again." And he never did, until the day he died—fifty years later.

Distinguishing Yourself from Your Addiction

Have you ever been in the middle of a heated debate with someone, and halfway into your righteous, irrefutable argument, you realize in a flash that you are wrong? What do you do? If you're like most people, you'll finish the sentence the way you started it. For some reason, that instant of clarity just isn't enough to stop you in your tracks or make you shift gears. Still, you heard it—that gentle, compelling voice that sends you signals and information from some deep, still place in your mind—"you're wrong."

This voice seems to assert itself out of nowhere. It's like a whisper that has the power to break through a trance, or like a flash of lightning that exposes the edge of a cliff just before you step off. Whatever you call this voice—God, conscience, life force, inner child, authentic (or true) self, wise mind, instinct—it presents you with a window of opportunity to exercise your options, even when you feel like you're riding a rocket train to hell.

As you know, hearing that voice and heeding it are two different things. In the first chapter, we witnessed Rose reject and ignore that voice time and again. The voice is just not as compelling or demanding as the surface noise: the repetitive, negative chatter that has created well-worn grooves in your mind and body—your addictive cravings, compulsions, and habits. Perhaps you've experienced being zoned out in front of the TV or the computer, deeply engrossed in the flickering images and barrage of junk information, when out of nowhere a window opens up in your mind and a vista of options appears: "I should get up and walk the dog . . . pick berries . . .

call a friend . . . read a book." You've probably heard some variation of this old joke: *I suddenly got the urge to exercise, so I sat down and waited for it to pass.* When that window of opportunity opens, we tend to do just that: hang tight and then reimmerse ourselves in the trance.

It can feel as if there are two of you in your own mind: One of "you" is being led around by the nose, while the other is watching. One is in thrall to urges, battered by incessant demoralizing beliefs and thoughts, including that your addiction is irresistible, while the other looks on in wonder and protest. When you ask yourself, "What the hell am I doing?"—a question everyone asks from time to time—this is one of your selves questioning the other. This invisible interchange *proves* that you are *not* your addiction.

Everyone knows such conflicts. No one is in perfect alignment with their best instincts or values all the time. But many people are able to correct course to improve their alignment either naturally or intentionally. Consider overworked parents who put in long hours in order to support their families, but who eventually realize that the time they spend away from home and family betrays their primary purpose. So they make changes in their work schedules in order to honor what they truly value: spending time together as a family.

What is unique when you are addicted, however, is that the hammering voices, urges, and cravings *overwhelm* your deeper voice. You have built a barrier, a screen, in the channel of communication, and continuing to act on your addiction serves to reinforce this blockage. Being addicted is like existing in a frantic state of patching and mending the screen between your authentic self and your addicted self. It's as if that screen separating your two selves were the only thing keeping you alive. But what's keeping you alive is your authentic self. The good news is that, no matter how much patching you do on the screen, the voice of your authentic self can't be extinguished. It remains unaffected by the racket your addicted self is making and continues to press to escape from behind the screen.

If you have ever enjoyed playing in the ocean, then you know what to do when a huge wave is about to pummel you: You dive under it, because the water below remains still, as if nothing is happening under the tumult. It is amazing how peaceful it is down there when that powerful force is crashing overhead. If you were the ocean, your true self would reside in the calm waters under the waves.

These truths about the dual self, the true self, the trance, and conflicting inner voices are timeless. Ancient spiritual traditions from all over the world, along with modern psychology, continually return to this phenomenon. In this chapter, I introduce you to your two selves in a very basic way, which you can filter through your religious faith or understand as simply a mechanism of human nature, as you see fit. I bring these concepts into the realm of addiction because they are on stark display wherever an addiction has staked its claim. It may help to think of the two voices—addiction and true self—as your two hands. Addiction is like the dominant arm and side of your body that respond preemptively to the tasks confronting you. The process of overcoming addiction is like deliberately developing the skill and strength in your other arm so that it can instead assert control. As your true self becomes stronger and more adept, your addiction loosens its grip, allowing your true self to take charge.

At this moment you may have some very negative beliefs about yourself. You may believe that your true self is somehow corrupted or deviant. You may think that you simply do not have an identity outside your addiction—that you are not distinct from it. You may believe that you have behaved in ways that disqualify you from positive participation in society, or that any engagement with the world beyond your addiction is a tedious masquerade. I acknowledge those beliefs and feelings now as you venture into this chapter; I will not direct you to ignore them or get over them. The purpose of this chapter is to guide you toward an understanding of this inner dynamic, to help you recognize the different voices that are competing for your attention, and to teach you how to choose where you place your attention, which voice you heed. I will also offer you exercises and practices that will help you differentiate one voice from another. You can start the exercises immediately—at least contemplate those listed at the end of the chapter.

Moments of Grace

I've discussed how 12-step recovery and its proponents view addiction as "self-will run riot"; this book takes the opposite view: Authentic free will that springs from your own already healthy core is the engine of your recovery from addiction.

Look at it this way: the very act of seeking addiction treatment—indeed, reading this book!—is evidence that your healthy life force has asserted itself. You made a decision based on your best instincts and desires for wellness and acted on them. This simple, obvious truth undermines the foundation of the standard recovery model, which requires you to embrace the idea that you will always make self-destructive decisions when left to your own devices. So let's step briskly over this recovery mythology to explore how you can begin deliberately moving in the direction of true recovery.

Instead, let's think about *your power to control your destiny, your mindfulness.* To remind you, as I said in the introduction: mindfulness—which is both a Buddhist and a psychological concept[1]—is the ability to focus your attention on the present moment. The benefits of mindfulness are being actively pursued in medicine for a range of medical and psychological conditions.[2] But mindfulness is particularly relevant to addiction. Being fully aware of and noticing what you're doing strengthens your ability to surface the key elements of your addiction—your motivation, your situation, your needs, and your ability to make alternative choices. You can improve this ability as you can any mental or physical capacity, by learning about and practicing it through mindfulness meditation, which brings your attention to your immediate sensations. I provide mindfulness meditations throughout this book, beginning with a basic mindfulness meditation primer, following in the exercises with a description of "user-friendly mindfulness meditation" that you can practice by choosing meditation options that feel right for you and your situation.

The idea of mindfulness as living in the present can be oversimplified as "living for the now," as in "We're all gonna die, so let's get drunk (stoned)." On the contrary, the balancing perspective of psychological mindfulness is consideration of how what you're doing impacts your life now and going forward. Mindfulness is awareness of the full reality in which you are situated, not a blocking out of awareness.

Think of a moment recently when you were about to mindlessly light a cigarette or pour a drink or eat some chips or place a bet. Have you ever paused in this moment? When, just for a second, it seemed as if you were at a crossroad? *Why am I doing this? I don't have to do this. I don't want to do this.* Perhaps you looked ahead to the consequences, the impact the addictive action would have on the rest of your life, and your resulting feelings (shame, etc.). But, then, perhaps you automatically repressed these thoughts and continued with what you were doing. After all, there are also consequences to taking the road less traveled, the non-addictive choice: You will have to acknowledge your responsibility, which is often painful. You will have to acknowledge your power, as well, which can be overwhelming. You will have to find something else to do with the time you might have spent lost in addictive behavior. You will have to feel whatever difficult emotions you were about to suppress: boredom, grief, or fear. You will have to face the responsibility for the choices you have made or avoided, like strained family relationships or financial or health problems that are a result of your addiction. And, if you listen to that voice just once, won't it prevent you from ever being able to pursue your addiction in peace?

The pause can be a pivotal moment—it offers the chance for a shift in balance, when your deepest self breaks through the haze of your addiction, interrupting the momentum that often seems beyond your control. Recall from Rose's story how she would experience a moment of revulsion and conflict every time she injected herself. When you pause this way you are being presented with an opportunity to honor your true self. It's a *moment of grace*.

The word "grace" has many connotations, both religious and secular. In *Recover!*, grace describes those moments when you hear your true voice. In these terms, a moment of grace is the sudden awareness that you are at a pivotal point; it is a vision of your ideal life, an opportunity to make a decision and act with free will, to pursue your true, healthy motivations. A moment of grace is a period or place in which you present yourself with options, when the addictive busywork, the repetitive patchwork of your life, is suspended and you see yourself from a clear vantage point—not from the outside, but from the inside, from the calm under the waves. It's a chance to move your life scales out of the balance they are now in—to tip them and shift the weight to the *positive, healthy arm of the scale*.

These moments may seem to happen accidentally, as they did for Rose and Ozzie. For Rose, it occurred when she dwelled on the impact of missing her daughter's birthday party. It made her feel as though she were no longer her child's mother. As for Ozzie, hadn't he noticed his nicotine-stained hands any time in the previous twenty-five years before deciding to quit smoking that day at lunch? Or Dori, in Chapter 2, who quit drinking when she saw several haggard women barflies and imagined herself as one of them—hadn't she ever seen the signs of aging due to her heavy drinking and smoking before she reached her thirties? What caused all of them to see themselves as though from their mind's eye?

Whether you choose to act on any given insight—to make changes—may also seem inexplicable. You might ask yourself why Rose didn't quit *in the first place*, rather than miss her daughter's birthday party, or why she didn't avoid all of the steps that *led up* to that moment. Why did she have to stew on that experience afterward—one which, after all, she chose? It seems as though she needed to experience that painful moment as a message from her own heart, even though she hadn't used similar previous internal communications to elevate herself. Instead, they had caused her to berate herself, giving her more reason to use.

While these moments can seem fleeting and illusory, The PERFECT Program helps you use them as the foundation of permanent changes you will make in your life. When your true self emerges, however briefly or quietly, this is your opening for change. As you learn to recognize and build on these instances, your core values and life purpose will become stronger, louder, more assertive, while your addiction becomes *less* compelling, *more* incompatible with what's important to you and, finally, *irrelevant*, indeed, offensive, to your life—as it did in the second half of Ozzie's life, and for Dori, who has become an advocate for people seeking to quit addictions on their own.

Shifting the Balance

Sometimes, the natural processes of maturing, taking on greater responsibilities, and finding meaning in life combine to make self-destructive behavior impossible. For example, an alcoholic might completely stop the dangerous practice of driving drunk once she becomes a mother. Now that her own children are in the back seat, she rejects that reckless behavior in her gut. The option of doing such a thing is permanently off the table, even if her addiction to alcohol persists. This mother experienced a significant natural righting of course when her behavior became incompatible with what she truly valued. This change in her driving habits might eventually provide her with the foundation to make further permanent changes in her life, including giving up her addiction, as becoming a parent does for innumerable addicts.

Many of us live in a state of conflict or despair, eaten up by the knowledge that we are violating our core values, but unable to find the commitment or will to change course. As you may know through personal experience, a moment of grace will not be illuminated by a sunbeam from heaven. It's usually fleeting, and comes hand in hand with self-recrimination. But its ambivalent nature does not mean that the choice won't eventually be clear, or that you do not have the power within yourself to change. Nor does it mean that this voice isn't already influencing you in positive ways, even if it is not strong enough to revolutionize your life in one fell swoop. Being able to recognize when your healthy self is asserting itself is the first step toward shifting the balance.

Perhaps Rose would have emerged from her trance sooner if she had been aware of the process occurring within and had been able to direct it intentionally. Remember when Rose began injecting meth? She felt acute shame and disgust each time she did so, which reinforced her belief that she was different—a completely lost soul who had to surrender herself—unworthy of attempting to live a productive life like a "normal" person. Mainstream recovery wisdom told her that she actually *was* different, so it's no wonder that she would immediately adopt such a hopeless perspective at times like this.

How much more empowering it would have been for Rose to recognize her inner turmoil as evidence of something positive about herself rather than as something broken!

The unease Rose felt when shuttling her daughter off so that she could be alone with her drug, which never failed to arouse her deepest values, caused her emotional discomfort because she was able to feel just how far off course she was. Awareness and understanding of this dynamic would have allowed her to see this discomfort as a positive sign, a signal that her behavior was betraying her truth. The *only* way for her to quell this dissonance was to change her behavior in line with her values.

Finding Your Mindfulness. Now that you are aware of your inner voice, you can try an experiment: The next time you find yourself pausing before or during an addictive behavior, turn your attention to that voice and notice the options it presents to you, while acknowledging the emotions you are experiencing. This is a simple act of mindfulness, in which you consciously—even if just briefly—extend the duration of that pause by focusing on it. Draw it out and sit with the discomfort as long as you can, even if you ultimately turn back to your addiction. Do this exercise whenever you have an opportunity.

Phil (whom we met in Chapter 2) had begun smoking at thirteen and had tried repeatedly to quit—succeeding for a few months two times, with a nicotine patch and nicotine gum, each time relapsing. At age sixty-nine, he awoke from his heart bypass operation, following his second heart attack, to see his lovely, thirty-six-year-old daughter Cynthia hovering over him. "Can you get me a cigarette, Cynthia darling?" he asked, as he had so many times before. "Daddy," Cynthia responded, "if you smoke another cigarette I'll never speak to you." Phil lived fourteen more years and, like Ozzie after his moment of truth, never smoked again.

Both Ozzie and Phil are confusing for those brain-hijacking theories of addiction I reviewed in Chapter 2. In one theory, addiction specialists explain how, once the body becomes accustomed to a certain cellular nicotine level, it is impossible for the person to tolerate falling below this level. So how could one sentence cure Phil and Ozzie? For these two addicts—safe within the social acceptance given smokers in their lifetimes—the crystallizing of their values by a seemingly stray comment in retrospect makes sense.

CASE: Wilson was born considerably later than Phil and Ozzie—almost three-quarters of a century later—although his life overlapped with both of theirs when *he* began smoking as a teenager. A painter, Wilson didn't fit the image many had of the carefree artist. He was conscientious and worked diligently both on his paintings and on jobs he held to put himself through school. In fact, Wilson tended to be anxious and to overworry his life.

So it seemed Marie, a carefree fellow artist he met, was a good match for him. Aside from their opposite dispositions, Wilson and Marie shared many values. They also both smoked. Then, suddenly, Marie quit (she had never been a heavy smoker). But Wilson persisted, even though Marie's example reminded him daily that he didn't really want to continue his addiction. As they reached their early thirties, the couple decided to have a child, and Marie became pregnant. Wilson quit smoking.

While talking on the phone to her mother in another city, Marie mentioned casually that Wilson had quit. Her mother exhaled a loud "*Thank*

God!" Marie responded, "I knew Wilson would never smoke after we started having children. Everyone knew he'd be a devoted dad."

Wilson, who was sitting nearby in their small apartment, heard his mother-in-law's first thankful prayer through the phone, but nothing more from her end. He shrugged inwardly. He was nonetheless proud that his wife had such confidence in him, which he had proved correct.

"How's your mom?" he asked Marie.

Ex-addicts like Ozzie and Phil can point to a precise pivotal moment of grace when a sudden realignment took place. Others' moments aren't so precise. Wilson's decision was a clear and necessary development in his life that he wouldn't ignore. Rose, on the other hand, circled back on her moment after she failed to heed it initially. Ultimately refusing to accept that she was no longer a mother—even as she hadn't been acting like one for some time—Rose finally rebelled against her addiction. The birthday party represented a flashing sign that she was crossing into territory where she refused to go. Wilson quit because he couldn't, in this day and age, imagine himself as a smoking father. Phil quit smoking when his daughter made him choose between her and his cigarettes. She spoke directly to his deepest self at just the right time and made an offer he couldn't refuse. Ozzie quit when a teasing comment from an acquaintance shifted his perspective, allowing him to see how his dependence on tobacco companies clashed with his pro-labor principles. Ozzie had never tried to quit before, unlike Phil, who had tried many times, and Wilson, who worried about quitting long before he did.

These examples demonstrate different ways people have aligned with their deeper selves. But all of these people, when they have overcome their addictions, have a reason that springs from a deep well of meaning within them. Reading these stories may make you worry, even despair, that *you* are different from these happy ex-addicts—that *your* addicted self is stronger, more insistent, unconquerable. "You," your addicted self whispers in your head, "are so far gone that even loving your child isn't enough," as it said to Rose. "What *is* the matter with you?" Perhaps you cannot think of *anything* that would give your life meaning or satisfaction beyond your addiction.

Mindfulness Reflection: Meet Your Addicted Self. If you are experiencing discouraging thoughts about yourself after reading these stories, please take the time now to acknowledge these difficult feelings and thoughts. There is no need to dwell on them, because we will address them fully in the next chapter. Accept and regard them with curiosity and the recognition that you will turn your complete attention to them soon.

For now, it is enough that you accept two things: (1) When you experience a "pause" in the momentum of your addiction, your inner wise mind is asserting itself; (2) When someone overcomes an addiction, it is because a shift in balance has occurred that aligns their choices with their deeply held values and purpose. And, before we go any further, you must keep this in mind—Ozzie and Phil became ex-addicts only after years of active addiction. Ozzie was heavily addicted for twenty-five years, Phil for five *decades*. Dori drank heavily for two decades, stunting her adult development. And Rose gave away her *child*. So you are not the worst addict we will encounter in *Recover!*.

That you can recover despite the length and severity of your addiction has been shown time and again by smokers and other addicts. Following the 1964 Surgeon General's Report labeling cigarettes as cancer-causing, it seemed like only the worst, most addicted smokers would continue their addictions. A National Cancer Institute monograph, *Those Who Continue to Smoke*,[3] asked, "Are [residual] smokers less likely to quit now than in the past?" What they found: "Surprisingly, none of the papers provides compelling evidence that this is the case." So, no matter how badly addicted you are, for no matter how long, you can quit. "Perhaps most provocative, however, are NHIS (National Health Interview Survey) data showing those aged 65 and over and 45 to 64 have the lowest rates of current smoking prevalence and highest quit ratios." That is, even when older people remain smokers after others have quit, they are *still* more likely to quit than younger smokers. I believe this is due to people's (yes, even longtime addicts') sense of their mortality.

Hitting Bottom?

Do Rose, Dori, Phil, Ozzie, and the other addicts whose lives we have glimpsed all demonstrate the phenomenon of "hitting bottom"? (Wilson clearly does not.) This is another piece of recovery mythology that says that only when addicts reach the absolute nadir in their lives can they possibly quit. Hitting bottom is supposed to be a do-or-die crossroad, a point at which things cannot get worse, so they have to get better. Often, people in the recovery world explain away an addict's failure to stay on the wagon by claiming that this person has not yet hit bottom—that they have to keep plunging powerlessly to ever-deepening depths of humiliation, danger, and self-betrayal. Wow! Can you see how this vision of recovery actually encourages the *pursuit* of greater degradation? Because it is only at the lowest point of existence, when the alternative is death, that you will finally surrender and work the steps. What a grim, terrifying scenario this is! It is also a complete fantasy, starting with Wilson and many addicts like him who simply refuse to go down that route.

"Hitting bottom" in the recovery industry is simply a term used to shift the goalposts. There is nothing scientific, or even anything specific, about it. "Bottom" cannot be defined or pinpointed. If you die in a gutter, without seeking recovery, it shows that you have a really "low bottom," that you just didn't get far enough down to reach out. And if you quit your addiction, even if nothing horribly bad has happened, then you have a "high bottom." And what about the many people for whom nothing in particular has actually happened when they recover—what "event" caused Ozzie, a shop steward and heavily addicted smoker, or Dori, an attractive woman and serious alcoholic, to quit?

Aside from exposing it as logical nonsense, I believe it is even more important to reject this crazy notion of hitting bottom on the grounds that it is irresponsible and dangerous. If you believe that you must hit bottom before you can recover, then you *have to* pursue the scorched-earth policy of self-destruction that can be fully demonstrated only by bankruptcy, homelessness, communicable diseases, driving accidents, rape, prostitution, prison, brain or liver damage. . . . In fact, when you think about it, unless you are dead, things can always get worse. And, that worse things await you if you don't quit is actually a helpful insight when you consider it from a non-12-step perspective. You may be mortified by your position or your behavior, but even from the depths of depravity, you can always descend even further.

Let's cut ourselves loose from this therapeutic nightmare. The truth is that as long as you can say to yourself *this is not what I want for myself*, recovery is always possible. However low down you are or are not, you can choose to extricate yourself from that mess just as readily as—more easily than—you can end up at the bottom of the dung heap with your last gasp of life. Because there is no such place as "the bottom." The directive to hit bottom is actually an instruction to *imagine* what for you would be the worst thing in your life, to plumb the dark pit of your soul. But it works only if you regard that image as an elevated moment of grace—a sign to look up instead of down. As sports psychologists teach people, you will head in the direction that you look *toward* and fulfill the goals you visualize for yourself.

> **In short:** *There is no reason you must find your lowest low in order to recover. You do not have to live your worst nightmare in order to discover what is truly important to you. You can start wherever you are.*

It is true that many people make a drastic change in their lives when they find themselves shocked or deeply ashamed of their own behavior. Sometimes, your first instinct is to suppress the pain by curling up and sinking deeper into your addiction. Other times, these feelings inspire a radical realignment. Rose, for instance, regularly received warning messages from outside (school, parents, work) as well as from within herself. Although, given the strong undertow of her cravings, she didn't act on these messages for some time, they nonetheless manifested in her as revulsion, regret, shame, and fear—and sometimes also as a promise to herself to quit or a brief feeling of inspiration and determination.

Rose did not hit bottom when she missed her daughter's party. Among her low moments, this doesn't stand out as the lowest. For instance, it couldn't be considered worse than sending her daughter to live with her parents, or beginning to inject meth, or watching herself deteriorate physically, or any of the other degrading episodes she had grown accustomed to. So why did a missed party trigger a shift, when having to make a choice between her addiction and her daughter hadn't been enough to make her change her course? If missing the party wasn't Rose's absolute, do-or-die bottom, then what was unique about that situation?

Rose's moment occurred when she perceived the difference between what she truly valued and where she was actually headed in a way she finally could not ignore. The missed party signaled a *person she would not let herself be*. Just as Ozzie could not be a capitalist stooge, or Wilson and Phil could not bear to see themselves as unloving fathers when that image inescapably presented itself. Or think how once, after one long bout of heavy drinking, Dori was hospitalized near death, and her mother lay in bed grasping her to say good-bye. But that didn't make Dori quit. Yet imagining an old-hag version of herself—the vain Dori exercised and dieted religiously—did. Likewise, having seen the dark place of a mother who abandoned her child, Rose couldn't ignore her most dearly held value in order to enter it. Or, more accurately, to enter it and to remain there. After all, whatever smoking signified to Ozzie about being captured by the capitalist system, he had been enslaved there twenty-five years before he leaped out one day like a cat from a hot tin roof.

Intentional Alignment

Aside from the fact that all the people in our stories demonstrate how overcoming addiction begins with an internal shift in balance, they appear to have another element in common: circumstance, even accident. Somehow—with Phil, or Ozzie, or Dori, or Rose—either they were shocked out of their addictive trance by a chance event or they experienced a sudden or subtle mental shift that they couldn't pinpoint. It is tempting to believe that none of these people had control over the positive changes in their lives any more than they had control over their addiction. And they are representative of a legion of people who have gone through similar experiences. It may seem that the shift was something that happened *to* them and that they were lucky or blessed by some mysterious force. You must remember, however, that the authentic self is not a foreign entity. It's not an elusive, unknowable presence. When people overcome their addictions, they are not transforming into completely different people. They are merely surfacing another side of themselves, an alternative persona, one that has been hidden and yet that represents their true, abiding self.

Being addicted means that you identify so strongly with your addiction, you are so consumed with the never-ending task of patching that flimsy screen that keeps your true self from emerging, that you have forgotten how to imagine yourself living without it. You would be empty inside or a complete stranger to yourself, someone without an identity or soul, you may now believe. *Recover!* and The PERFECT Program tell you: **This is not true.** The real you is, in fact, able to reassert itself and to take charge. He or she is the very familiar *you* who is reading these words on this page right now. And *that* you is not fundamentally, perpetually, or irrevocably an addict. The addicted you is disposable—may even be displaced while you read these words.

But it can be as hard for you to remove your addictive thinking and identity as it is to rid yourself of the addictive behavior—harder. They're probably making quite a racket in there, encouraged (as in Alan's case that begins Chapter 2) by popular misinterpretations of science—often spread in the recovery world or via media—that say you are unable to change. Like so many other ideas about yourself you harbor—"you can't do this; you have no authentic self; you're going to be fat forever; you are worse than Rose or anyone else; you'd never be happy if you couldn't hang out at bars with your friends; everyone secretly thinks you're weird . . . blah blah blah"—*these ideas are false.*

You know instinctively that Rose, Dori, Phil, and Ozzie did not lose an essential part of themselves when they abandoned their addictions. Rather, they grew more fully into who they truly are: within themselves, in relation to others, in connection to their worlds. Having now emerged from the cocoon of their addictions, they will not be *less* themselves for having emerged, for making this effort, and for eventually finding their perch in the real world (that is, one not colored by their drugs or addictive experiences). What made the transformations seem accidental or external in the cases presented was only these individuals' lack of awareness of the natural recovery process unfolding within them and of their power to manage it. But, now that *you* are aware of the inner dynamics at play, you can nurture this transformation in yourself. And you can start now, right where you are, by learning to focus on the signals from your core and to distinguish them from the cravings and urges that have trapped you until now.

Recall the ocean surf analogy earlier in this chapter and imagine yourself in the calm deep water under the waves. The force and spectacle of the waves overhead is very much like your addiction—rushing and crashing over everything in its path—but always in flux, changing and shifting. A wave has no permanence, and neither does your addiction. Underneath the waves, where your life is rich and abundant, is the deep calm in which you reside. Of course, you cannot stop the waves, but you can learn to shift your focus away from the surface turmoil. The mindfulness meditation exercise at the end of this chapter is a technique you will use to sharpen your underwater senses and begin to recognize your real voice from deep down within you. It will also allow you to recognize that the negative voices—the urges, cravings, and the vicious stories we tell about ourselves—lack permanence. Just like a wave. Yes, they are powerful and potentially destructive, just like waves, but they are just as transitory and ephemeral.

Moving Forward: Putting Mindfulness into Action

In this chapter, you have gathered some information that you can use as you continue your journey to true recovery. Now, when you pause to ask yourself, "What the hell am I doing?," you will recognize that as a moment of grace, a communication from yourself and an interlude filled with possibility. Simply turning your attention to that voice will bring you into contact with your core, sharpen your interior senses, and begin the conscious shift of your life's balance. This is the process of mindfulness in recovery. Beginning a daily mindfulness meditation practice is a gentle way for you to initiate the process of natural recovery by learning to harness your free will. *Mindfulness skills will also be your bedrock of relapse prevention.*

Maybe you still believe that change isn't possible for you, that your addiction is intractable, or even that you don't deserve a full life. That is okay. For now, focus only on distinguishing the competing voices within and practice the following exercises. In the next chapter, we will explore these negative beliefs about yourself and guide you to a place of self-acceptance.

Mindfulness and addiction

You may suspect that I emphasize the practice of mindfulness meditation throughout The PERFECT Program in order to take advantage of the mindfulness craze. As mindfulness has come to the fore in recent years, there are now manuals for mindfulness for just about everything people want to do: selling, money management, medicine, marriage, parenting, exercise, eating, pet ownership, even sewing. Clearly, mindfulness is a trend. But it is also a deep and powerful practice that has been passed down for thousands of years. And, as this chapter makes clear, it speaks directly to and combats the essential mechanism in addiction.

Addiction is the mindless and relentless chasing of superficial urges and compulsions, a desperate grasping at fleeting satisfaction; mindfulness is its perfect, natural opposite and antidote. In fact, that is exactly what it was meant to achieve. Mindfulness is a respite from craving that you create through the practice of bringing your full awareness into the present moment, rather than allowing yourself to be led mindlessly by force of habit. The usefulness of the Marlatt team's mindfulness-based approach to relapse prevention illustrates this principle.[4] Mindfulness may be the buzzword *du jour*, but for combating addiction it is a central, crucial practice. Mindfulness has proven especially useful in dealing with binge eating,[5] which appears both in regard to obesity and to eating disorders such as anorexia and bulimia.[6]

As I have written: "Addiction is the search for emotional satisfaction—for a sense of security, a sense of being loved, even a sense of control over life. But the gratification is temporary and illusory, and the behavior results instead in greater self-disgust, reduced psychological security, and poorer coping ability. That's what all addictions have in common."[7] There is no place where this cycle is clearer than in the case of binge eating. Binge eating points clearly to the nature of the addictive experience as a self-feeding negative relationship to an object, activity, or involvement. As one woman spoke of coalescing obese binge eaters and those with eating disorders: "The problem [for either the anorexic or bulimic, or the obese, binge eater] is not the food; the problems are the issues in your life, and you turn to food because you can't handle them."

As the foundation of The PERFECT Program, developing your mindfulness practice is key. So, if the very thought of meditation makes you groan in anticipation of excruciating tedium, well . . . get that groan out of your system now. Go ahead—groan!

Done? Then let's get started!

Meditation

Basic Mindfulness Meditation

It is often difficult for people with addictions to meditate. The idea of just sitting with yourself for any length of time can seem overwhelming, especially when you are preoccupied with patching your addictive screen to hide your real self. This meditation is thus an exercise of your free will, as well as a technique for making contact with your core self.

Find a quiet place, where you know you will be undisturbed, and a place to sit, either on a chair, a cushion, or on the floor. Don't lie down: You want to be in a state of relaxed attention, not fall asleep. Set a timer for ten minutes (if ten seems overwhelming, start with five and work up to ten). Find a comfortable position, rest your hands on your lap, close your eyes, and relax every muscle. Focus your attention on each part of your body and release the tension there. When you are relaxed, turn your attention to your breathing: listen to the sound of your breath, notice the duration of each breath, the sensation of taking air into your lungs. If it helps you to focus, you can think "in breath" and "out breath." As you do this, thoughts and emotions will enter your mind, some random, some uncomfortable. When this happens, acknowledge them, notice them, and release them, and then deliberately shift your attention back to your breathing.

There is no right way to meditate, and no particular experience you should have. It's important to remember that, even if you spent the whole time fidgeting and distracted, that is not wrong. That was simply your experience; you are learning the skill of sitting with uncomfortable feelings. You are not obligated to act on every urge or thought that presents itself to you. Remember that no one can block out all thoughts and feelings, so don't make that your goal. You cannot control what thoughts come into your mind. Notice how fluid these thoughts and feelings are, how they come and go, and how you can turn your attention away from them. You cannot stop them from coming, but you can consciously control where you place your attention. With daily practice, you will find it ever easier to turn your awareness where you choose to and let the waves of thoughts and feelings flow over you and away.

Tips:

- Create a permanent space in your home for meditation, where you will be comfortable and undisturbed by noise or clutter.
- Get an egg timer or an alarm with a gentle chime—not your cell phone timer; your phone might ring.
- Turn off the ringer on your phone.
- Set a regular time every day for meditation, when you know you will be alert.

- Challenge yourself to increase your meditation time weekly by five minutes. Set a goal of at least thirty minutes.
- Find a meditation center or group in your neighborhood.

Mindfulness Variation: You can bring mindfulness practice into your everyday life. Whenever you think of it, stop and bring your full presence to whatever you are doing. For instance, if you are washing dishes, challenge yourself to notice as many details as you can about the activity: How do the suds feel? What do they look like? What temperature is the water? How do you feel about doing the dishes? Or focus inward—on your mind and your body (instead of listening to your iPod)—while you exercise. Remain mindful as long as possible, and see if you can extend these periods of full awareness.

Relapse Prevention Starts Now: Research is demonstrating the effectiveness of mindfulness techniques in relapse prevention. Studies conducted at the University of Washington, for instance, report a significant decrease in relapse as well as cravings in participants who employ mindfulness-based practices compared to those who receive "treatment as usual."[8] Starting a mindfulness meditation practice now will provide you with a strong foundation for maintaining your success, giving you a powerful skill that will aid in both preventing relapse and correcting course in the event that you do relapse.

Exercises

Activating Your Free Will: Acting with free will is the ability to align your choices and behaviors with what is truly important to you. Simple enough in theory, but it takes deliberate practice. Once you have the ability to see your addictive urges for what they are and to distinguish them from your healthy core self, you can begin to choose where to focus. In other words, you can train your free will to take over. Let's begin by committing to use this powerful anti-addiction tool in your daily life:

S.P.O.T.

- **See:** When you have an addictive urge, *see* it for what it is. Mindfully appraise the feeling as addiction, distinct from the conscious presence that you are using to recognize it. There is the urge, and there is you acting as witness to the urge. Say, "This is an addictive urge."

- **Pause:** Allow yourself to sit with your addictive urge, to experience the uncomfortable feelings, or even the emotional pain that results from not immediately acting on your craving. Set a time frame for yourself and commit to not acting on this urge—say, thirty minutes to start. Or if that's too difficult, start smaller and work your way up.
- **Override:** While you are waiting it out, engage yourself in a life-affirming activity that you know will bring you some sense of accomplishment or satisfaction. Make a list of things you can do at a moment's notice to override your addictive urge (there are some suggestions for you in the "Triage" chapter on page 241).
- **Track:** Keep track of your S.P.O.T. progress: record how long you were able to Pause and what you did to Override your addictive urge. Focus only on your successes and on what worked for you. Do not berate yourself if you succumbed. Remember, you are strengthening your "weaker hand," and that takes effort, time, and patience.

Journal Exercises

Your Moments of Grace: Can you identify any recent instances in which you experienced a "pause" in your addictive behavior? Perhaps you were about to indulge your addiction and were overcome with a feeling of tedium or repulsion. Maybe you extinguished a half-smoked cigarette out of a sudden feeling that you were wasting your time or making yourself sick. Perhaps you put down a cream puff or morning pastry by thinking, "Is this really something I like?" Or you may have looked at your friends drinking or smoking weed at a party and considered, "Maybe I'll just sit out this shift." Write about these instances in as much detail as you can recall, extending for as long as you held out against your addictive urges. If you did relent and indulge, include the thoughts or feelings that eventually led you to persist in your addictive behavior. Try to answer these questions:

- What did that moment of grace communicate to you? How did it present itself? As a feeling? A thought? An image? Was it a negative idea or image of the activity, or a positive one of what might be?
- How long did it last? How did it make you feel?

If you dismissed it and continued to pursue your addiction, write about what you said to yourself, or how you suppressed that inner voice.

Telling a New Story: Choose one of the moments of grace you wrote about in the last exercise and tell the story again, only this time give it a different ending. Write a new story about yourself: Imagine that you honored that voice and chose not to pursue the addiction. What would you have chosen to do instead? What would you have accomplished? Explore your new story in as much detail as you can. It is like writing a work of fiction with you at the center, except that "fiction" is the real you.

Yoga and Mindfulness

Yoga offers many of the same benefits as meditation—indeed, many yoga classes and videos begin and/or end with brief meditations. I practice yoga—which I summarize as stretching and breathing. As in meditation, the centering focus of all activity is on your breath, along with a deep awareness of your body. For people inclined to physical exertion and for whom the restful poses of meditation don't come naturally, yoga can be a better route to mindfulness.

Introducing yoga into your routine will broaden and deepen your experience with mindful awareness. Of course, yoga is good exercise and can help you become stronger and more limber. But it has benefits beyond exercise. Just as with meditation, yoga requires you to bring your awareness fully into the present moment. As with meditation, the benefits are in simply doing it, at any level of proficiency. As you take your body into new positions, you may be aware of uncomfortable sensations or emotions, but turning your curious attention to these feelings is part of the exercise. Like meditation, yoga offers a balancing experience to your day in which you engage your mind, body, breathing, and your setting simultaneously, in the moment.

If you haven't done yoga or don't know how to begin a practice, it is an easy activity to access. Classes are readily available, either privately or at no added cost at Y's, health clubs, or other community venues. Gaiam (www.gaiam.com), Amazon, and many other sites offer numerous yoga videos, including many for beginners, some of which may be available at your library. Among many books you can find on yoga is *Moving Toward Balance: 8 Weeks of Yoga with Rodney Yee.* Yee guides you through a home-based yoga practice while delving into the mind and body benefits of this practice, a valuable addition to your mindfulness tools.

Other Mind-Body Programs

There are many varieties of mind-body learning aside from yoga, some almost as well known (including tai chi, Pilates). Any of these is worth exploring, even though I can't go into detail about them here. Another form of such movement/meditation is the Feldenkrais Method. Feldenkrais emphasizes mindful self-awareness, including visualization, in order to relearn common motions to improve performance, encourage ease and pleasure of movement and function, and reduce pain and injury. Feldenkrais involves instruction, but is also self-directed and non-routinized, relying on the person's creativity and experience. It is a gentle practice that proceeds in gradual increments. Typical Feldenkrais advisories are to be aware when practicing so as to avoid discomfort, to enjoy the practice, and to integrate new learning with everyday living and movement. You may find instruction and classes at the Feldenkrais Method website (www.feldenkrais.com).

User-Friendly Mindfulness Meditation

This additional meditation section reviews the basic meditation approach I described above, but in a more general and open way, to allow you to tailor your meditation practice as you see fit and to feel comfortable exploring your options.

The heart of mindfulness meditation practice is in willfully directing your attention to the present moment and your feelings and sensations within it. You can find your own way of achieving that experience. This will be a self-directed practice, so experiment with approaches to meditation to find what works best for you. Typically, people sit on a cushion with their legs crossed and backs erect. Your ambition might be to levitate six inches off the ground in a perfect lotus position, but (since that is only for advanced students) you may be most comfortable sitting in a straight-backed chair. Similarly, you may find it easier to keep your eyes softly focused on a candle flame than to keep your eyes closed (especially if you have a tendency to sink into a torpor when you meditate). You may want to rest your hands on your knees, palms up, relaxed and open, or you may feel more secure with your fingers touching your thumbs, palms down on your knees, or softly folded in your lap, or together at your heart. Whatever position you choose, notice how it makes you feel, what sensations or feelings each position creates for you.

The purpose of mindfulness meditation is not to empty your mind, to be clear of all thoughts. In fact, there is no state of mind you must strive to achieve, so that when you're finished you know whether or not you have been successful. Simply *doing* it is success. What will you be doing, then, exactly? You will be paying curious, nonjudgmental attention to whatever comes up, while intentionally directing and redirecting your mind to remain fully in the present. That is it. Here's the nuance: The practice is in continually and deliberately reinhabiting the present moment, not in trying to force yourself to remain in the present moment.

Think of your mind as a playful puppy that will chase after every squirrel or ball that crosses his path. It is in the puppy's nature to romp and chase. However, just because it is in his nature does not mean that his whims should always rule the roost. He must be trained to return to you when you call him, otherwise he might carelessly (mindlessly) chase a cat out into the road. As he matures into an adult dog, you don't want him to stop playing or protecting his territory, but you do want to make sure that you are the one in charge. As his master, you can call him back to your side when necessary.

You are not trying to prevent your mind from wandering or chasing after shiny objects. That's what our minds do. You simply want to train your mind to come when called. Traditionally, mindfulness practice begins by focusing your attention on your breath. It is the most convenient, ever-present touchstone—a bridge between the inner and outer landscapes you inhabit at every moment. Turning your attention to your breath is easy, because it is always there and you can always find it. There are a few ways of keeping your attention focused on your breath. You may, for instance, say to yourself (either silently or out loud), "In breath.

Out breath." You might also count your breaths. Count to ten, then start again—and again. If your mind wanders, start again. No judgment. Or, you might vocalize with each breath. You may know about chanting "Om," which is an option, as is simply making a sound that feels right to you as you breathe out.

Alternately, you may want to focus your attention on a part of your body or inner landscape that feels good or neutral. Or, use the sound of your refrigerator humming as your home base, if that works. You might choose to use a visual touchstone, either physical (like that candle flame) or by keeping your eyes closed and focusing on the spot between and just above your eyebrows. Some people see light or color there. In order to remind yourself to bring your attention back to the present, you can set a gentle chime to sound every ten or fifteen minutes. Or listen to a guided mindfulness meditation, which you can download from the Internet or purchase as a recording. If you find it difficult to sit, or are overcome with restlessness and do not have the tolerance for it yet, you may practice walking meditation. In walking meditation, you focus your attention on movement: your steps, your active muscles, your gait. Walk with intention, taking deliberate steps. And when you find your mind wandering, acknowledge it, and turn your attention back to your walking. The variations are endless, so to ensure consistent practice, take time to figure out what works best for you. The only correct way to practice mindfulness meditation is *your* way. As long as you are doing it, you are doing it right.

Meditation options

Here are some options to help guide you to a meditation practice that works best for you. Each option will generate different feelings or call different thoughts to mind. Bring your mindful attention to these feelings and thoughts. For instance, does sitting on a cushion make you feel more grounded than sitting on a chair? Or does sitting on a chair allow you to remain more alert? Does keeping your eyes closed make you feel disoriented, while keeping your eyes focused on a flame helps you feel more connected to your environment? Remember, as you continue your practice, these options will remain fluid. What makes you feel insecure one day may make you feel exhilarated the next. Today, you might need walking meditation; tomorrow, you might be willing to sit still and explore your restlessness.

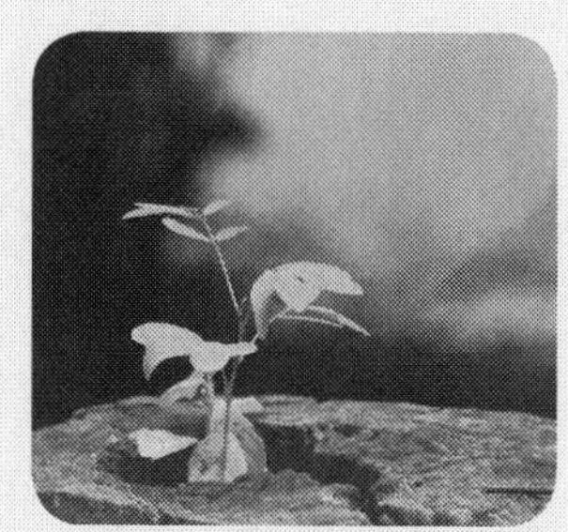

Location:
- Indoor meditation spot
- Altar
- Outside
- Walking (inside or outside)
- Meditation hall
- Other____________________________

Sitting Options:
- Floor
- Cushion on the floor
- Crossed legs
- Lotus position
- Chair
- Other ____________________________

Hand Position:
- Palms down, on your knees or lap
- Palms up, on your knees or lap
- Fingers touching thumb, on your knees or lap
- Hands at your sides or touching the floor
- Palms pressed together, at your heart center
- Other ____________________________

Mindfulness Touchstone (Home Base for Your Attention):
- Breath
- Chant, "Om" or other vocalization
- Physical sensation
- Emotional feeling
- Craving or urge (see Chapter 7)
- Physical object
- Inner visual image
- An intention
- Other____________________________

Guidance:
- None
- Recorded guided meditation
- Chimes at intervals
- Meditation class or group
- Other____________________________

CHAPTER 5

Embrace

Self-acceptance and forgiveness—Learning to love yourself

CHAPTER GOALS

- To balance mindfulness with compassion
- To make self-acceptance a new habit of mind
- To draw a distinction between your true self and your addiction
- To understand and practice forgiveness, of yourself and others

Purpose: It may seem that mindfulness implies stark introspection, requiring you to see all your flaws with brutal clarity. In other words, it could be yet another tool you can use to beat yourself up. But clarity of perception is logically tempered by self-acceptance. It simply makes sense for you to recognize that you are a worthy and complete person, entitled to fulfillment, opportunity, and love. With this realization in place, your self-examination will be balanced—both accurate and compassionate—which will make it effective. The purpose of this chapter is to guide you toward self-acceptance and its sister cognitive emotion, forgiveness—of yourself and others. With the joint tracks of mindfulness and self-acceptance in place, you can readily go forward with your PERFECT Program.

The Weight of Negativity

It may be human nature to suspect the worst about ourselves. Sometimes this impulse achieves pathological levels, as it does with people who suffer from a condition called "body dysmorphia." Those afflicted believe themselves to be so physically grotesque that they have no right to even walk outside as normal human beings do. They are unable to look in the mirror without feeling profound self-hatred, seeing shocking deformity and ugliness, even though their appearance is perfectly normal, or even beautiful, to those around them—especially those who see the whole person, inside and out. Think, for instance, of dangerously malnourished anorexics who believe themselves to be obese, exploring their bodies with microscopic attention to this pocket of fat or that small curve. When they look at themselves, all they can see are these magnified imperfections—they live a life of vigilance, self-denial, and self-debasement, trying to correct their overwhelming flaws, or they hide themselves away altogether.

Maia Szalavitz notes, "Being ashamed of drinking prompts relapse, not recovery."[1] In a study in which alcoholics were videoed reviewing their bad drinking episodes, when they were followed up four months later, researchers found that their displays of physical shame (coded on a scale of their body language) in the first ten seconds directly predicted their likelihood of relapse: every added point they scored led to an average of eleven more drinks over the period of the study. Even alcoholics displaying moderate shame drank twenty more drinks than those who didn't convey shame. Furthermore, a review of the use of "humiliating, confrontational tactics, which attempt to induce shame" found that not one study over four decades supported this approach.[2] "The results add to a body of literature suggesting that widely used shaming and humiliating methods of treating alcohol and other drug problems—such as those seen on shows like *Celebrity Rehab*—are not only ineffective but also may be counterproductive."

Yet shame and humiliation are the fundamental emotional experiences encouraged in recovery! Step 1, that you are powerless, is described as "absolute humiliation" by AA.[3] *Self-acceptance is the defining difference between AA and The PERFECT Program.* This is the place where The PERFECT Program most clearly and meaningfully diverges from the dysfunctional, defeatist model that has been pushed on you and so many others as the American approach to addiction. After you and fellow

AA members "admitted we were powerless over alcohol" (or whatever you're addicted to: shopping, food, sex, gambling, painkillers), you must then have "Made a moral inventory" of your failures (step 4), "Admitted to God," yourself, and others these failures (step 5), made yourself "ready to have God remove all these defects of character" (step 6), begged "Him to remove our shortcomings" (step 7), and then have "Made a list of all persons we had harmed" (step 8).

Feeling uplifted and ready to recover about now? The research indicates not. What's worse, conventional recovery's fixation on character defects appeals to the powerful impulse we have to believe the worst about ourselves. But recovery thus motivated is not compatible with a fully realized sense of yourself. Think of an anorexic or bulimic who has to overcome her sense of worthlessness, along with her belief that she is ugly. Is the path to achieving peace of mind for girls and others with these feelings to constantly examine and apologize for their various imperfections, many unnoticeable or irrelevant or not their fault, like those just about every other human being has? In fact, thinking that way is the problem! It's impossible to expect a person to achieve wellness by focusing on his or her faults and mistakes. Perhaps this is why conventional recovery asserts that people must remain "in recovery" forever and continue to identify themselves as addicts, no matter how long they are sober. It is the AA worldview itself that actually makes your recovery so tenuous by imposing a *perpetual state of spiritual dysmorphia.*

CASE: Alexis was, at twenty-eight, a tall, willowy model. And she had developed a terribly damaging case of anorexia. While this condition could be laid at the feet of the modeling business, it was also true that she had never seen herself as attractive—a habit of mind that continued now even as she graced the covers of leading fashion magazines around the world.

As a child, Alexis was regarded as tall and gawky. Asked to name her chief characteristic today, Alexis would note her elongated nose, near-sightedness (she wore glasses at home), and the very slenderness that was her stock-in-trade—"I wish I were more feminine," she sighed. As a result, she rarely went to social events, where she never felt she fit the role of glamorous model she was expected to fill.

Alexis was also an extremely caring person. She clucked after the younger models (many of whom were still in their teens) like a mother hen. When she became involved in a charity to help feed African children, the organization's representative remarked with amazement, "She really cares!" rather than simply supporting the charity because her publicity agent told her she should. Particularly noticeable was her affinity for—love of—injured and mutilated children she met, whom she hugged as if they were her own.

If you asked Alexis, someone with a debilitating case of body dysmorphia, whether anyone else—like the starving and bruised children she encountered—deserved the kind of abuse she inflicted upon herself—like withholding nourishment and mocking their appearance—she would have turned on you like a tigress. Her whole being was devoted to making them feel accepted and loved. Her irate reaction would be similar if you asked her the question, "Should people with blemishes hide themselves?"

Alexis would loudly protest that the idea that people should be preoccupied with their physical imperfections is preposterous, degrading, and completely unhelpful for these children and for society. So why does she hide herself, obsessed with her own flaws, believing that she alone, among all imperfect people on earth, deserves to be judged harshly? It's clear that her torment is caused by her inability to view herself through a lens of compassion, like the one through which she is able to see distressed children. Framed this way, it is apparent how warped her perspective towards herself is. In fact, Alexis's greatest need is to overcome this self-loathing in order to cure her addictive eating disorder, as young women often do as they mature, since eating disorders appear primarily in teens and young adults.[4]

The distorted perspective an anorexic has on her outward physical appearance is like the one you may train on your inner being when you conclude that you are so innately, irredeemably damaged or abnormal that you can never engage in life as everyone else does. Think of Alexis, in whom this prejudice against herself is so obvious. Alexis could never see herself as being as beautiful, engaging, popular, and accomplished as other people saw her to be. So she rejected the compliments—"you've really been there for so many younger models"; "you've created communities for yourself in modeling and around the world that should make you proud"; "you are a beautiful person, inside and out, Alexis"—as she gazed at herself in the mirror with disappointment and even repugnance.

Accentuating the Positive

Recover!'s approach to overcoming addiction requires a radical shift away from the self-degrading examination of yourself and your life in order to enumerate all of your horrible traits and despicable acts. For instance, your recovery program may tell you that you are naturally self-centered and dishonest, that if you are left to your own devices you will always make poor choices, and that you are obligated to focus constantly on such "character defects" and misdeeds, then hold them up for public examination. The PERFECT Program replaces this demeaning practice, one that reinforces what may be your already irresistible impulse to pathologize and reject yourself. Instead, *Recover!* asks you to embrace yourself as already worthy, whole, and wise. Above all, you should realize, *addiction is not a core identity any more than is a flabby thigh or a crooked nose*. They are all superficial characteristics, not foundations on which to build your identity.

CASE: Letter from a man who relapsed after attending AA

I sincerely want to change my habits. I am totally aware that what I am doing is self-destructive.

However, as a person who has survived severe emotional and physical childhood abuse, I cannot or will not ever again admit I am powerless. In spite of it all I am a medical professional who devotes each day to ensuring that my severely disabled patients enjoy the highest quality of life. I also respect their right to choose what is the best course for them.

I have failed AA because I am unable to confess I am powerless. I have been told that since I am unwilling to surrender I may as well give up on being sober, that this is my addicted brain talking. I feel that they're telling me I have no worth. Saying I'm powerless and going to 90 meetings in 90 days only reinforces my feelings that I am a failure. In all honesty I feel bad enough about myself as is. If I give up on me, who is left to carry on?

AA veterans have told me this is denial. Am I in denial? I know I drink too much; that is why I came to AA. I do know that when I am happy and doing meaningful work I don't care about drinking at all. And I know that telling myself how rotten I am won't change anything for me. In fact, it makes things worse. Which may be why I bought and consumed a bottle of wine after my last meeting.

Is what I am being told right? Right now I am lost and miserable.

While AA certainly helps some people, this man is far from unique. Ken Anderson noted, "I have also seen many people whose drinking got worse while attending AA. I am one such person: During my time in AA, I nearly died of alcohol withdrawal."[5]

This man needs not to have his wavering self-image further undermined, but to have his strengths and positive life instincts encouraged, reinforced, and extended. Indeed, we all need that. Consider the last time someone gave you a heartfelt compliment. Did you reflexively deny it or brush it off, as if it would be dishonest or presumptuous to accept it? It seemingly takes an act of will to acknowledge as true an attribute, skill, or good act of yours. The impulse to view your positive qualities with some modesty is reasonable. But, then, you should be just as measured when it comes to your demons. Let someone point out some deep personality flaw that you have—meanness, insecurity, bad faith, fear—and you will likely burrow into your cave and reflect on that insult endlessly. You almost certainly take it much more to heart than you would any praise that someone offers you. Why should insults affect you so much more than compliments? Regardless of the reasons behind this disparity, *your task for overcoming addiction is to find a way of perceiving in yourself what is right and good at least as readily as you reflect on your flaws and errors.* When you identify these positive qualities, you can't rule them out as insignificant exceptions (as Alexis did her charity work and generosity) while regarding your negative ones as being the real, permanent you. Maintaining some balance is only fair!

CASE: Have you ever noticed how hard it is for people to accept compliments?

At forty, Jack had never settled into a niche in life. Then he began working at a dog grooming service, making appointments, looking after dogs before their owners arrived, and taking payments. Jack had found

Nirvana! He was great with customers, loved animals and had a gift for handling them, and was as reliable and punctual as his boss had ever found an employee to be. As a result, she gave Jack more and more responsibility managing the business.

Susan, who brought her dog for grooming regularly, appreciated Jack's care, skill, and attention with her pet and with her. "Jack, I just so like bringing my dog here. You really seem to love your job!"

"That's because Elaine is the best boss I've ever had," Jack enthused. "She changed my life."

As it happened, Elaine was in the shop at the time. "That's because you don't see me at home, where I'm a real ______."

Susan had seen people deflect compliments hundreds, thousands of times. (She did so herself, she later reflected.) But this time, the phenomenon struck her. "Elaine," she blurted out, "Jack just said you changed his life, and you slough off his feelings as though they meant nothing!"

Exercise 1, Part 1

Before you read further, open your journal and make three columns. Title the first column, "I want to overcome my addiction because. . . ." Underneath that heading, list as many answers to that question as you can. Then continue reading. You'll find Part 2 of this exercise on page 111.

The shift in perspective The PERFECT Program requires is not simply from being all-out negative to uncritically positive. Believing the worst about yourself is unrealistic—but it's not any more realistic (or possible) simply to believe only the best about yourself and that everything is hunky dory. Balance requires avoiding *both* a microscopic scrutiny of your personal defects *and its opposite*, a silly Stuart Smalley self-affirmation ("I'm good enough; I'm smart enough; and doggone it, people like me"). A balanced view of yourself sees you as a complete, fundamentally sound person, one with both positive and negative aspects, neither of which define, support, or detract from your fundamental worth as a human being. It's like the difference in perspective between trying to make out the dirty pattern on the linoleum of an aged kitchen floor and looking at the whole planet from space. Self-acceptance is looking at yourself from the more complete, and therefore more forgiving, perspective of space.

In the previous "Pause" chapter, we introduced you to the practice of bringing your full awareness into the present moment. Mindfulness is a simple and powerful anti-addiction tool that serves you in several ways: It hones your ability to listen to your inner voice, your sound instincts. Mindfulness teaches you to distinguish between your life force and the temporary feelings, cravings, desires, and compulsions of addiction. It gives you the mental distance and room to note and explore where these uncomfortable feelings are coming from without having to act on them. It helps you develop the skill of sitting out these onrushing feelings without being swept away by them. In short, mindfulness is full presence and clarity. But mindfulness alone is not enough to free you from addiction. Self-acceptance—compassion for yourself as well as others—is an equal partner in this endeavor.

In the last chapter I promised to address the pessimism and discouragement you may feel about your ability to overcome addiction. You may believe, for instance:

- I am different from normal people. I don't have what it takes to beat my addiction. I have no identity outside of my addiction. My addiction is worse than anyone else's.
- I am *incapable* of creating a meaningful or fulfilling life. I am inherently deficient. I can't learn new skills or how to change.
- I do not *deserve* a meaningful or fulfilling life.
- I don't know how to act properly. No one has treated others as badly as I have. I have committed worse acts (sins) than everyone else.
- The good things in life are for other people.

Beliefs like these hurt you because you can feel right, and even noble, thinking the worst of yourself, as if you were simply being realistic about your limitations—that you are facing the cold facts. Since no one knows you like you do, hearing from strangers like me that you're not as bad as you think you are won't persuade you. The most difficult part of your journey to wellness will be loosening the grip these beliefs have on you and replacing them with positive, self-accepting ones.

Exercise 1, Part 2

Revisit your answers to the question, "I want to recover from addiction because . . ." and see if you can recognize the extent of your negative critiques of yourself. For example, "I want to recover from addiction because I am a terrible parent."

What's Really Wrong with You?

Feeling that you are off the grid in some way is common not only for addicts, but for everyone, even those who seem to have it all. But addicts have an added blanket of self-contempt to contend with, because addiction often goes hand-in-hand with estrangement, deception, inner conflict, and shame. To take one example, you will typically hear addicts despair of their discomfort and lack of confidence in new social situations, as if their awkwardness is unique to them as addicts (this may be a feeling you know well yourself). Many explain they used drugs or drank initially in order to relax in social situations.

It's true that addicts and alcoholics can feel out of place in social situations. But only the rare social butterfly doesn't feel uncomfortable around new people—put another way, nearly everyone feels more comfortable in familiar settings with people they know. True, if you have spent a lifetime quelling your social anxiety with an addiction, you may have built quite a structure on this common insecurity, because you haven't had the opportunity to develop healthier ways of coping. But these experiences nonetheless fall well within the normal spectrum of human experience. They are not unique to you and other addicts, and it isn't true that you can *never* remedy these feelings. You *can* change such responses by exposing yourself to new social environments in new ways.

Even the most progressive addiction experts in the field, those who reject the destructive aspects of recovery culture, seem unable to shake the habit of searching for underlying pathologies common to addicts. The fact that the field can't settle on what your real problem is should give you pause: Is it childhood trauma? Or has your brain chemistry gone haywire? Or maybe you lack the inherited chemical means to process alcohol (this is one that may strike entire races!).[6] You can find a whole laundry list of root causes. Perhaps you were abandoned as a child. Perhaps you were overly attached to your mother. Could be you have no impulse control or an inability to delay gratification. Maybe you can't process sugar or white bread or are deficient in amino acids. The list is endless, especially when these experts start mixing and matching. There's no doubt you can find one or more of these theories that apply to you.

What makes this approach so compelling is that it homes in on addicts' urges to embrace any evidence supporting their deeply held belief that there is something fundamentally wrong with them. Now, at last, you have an explanation for your problems; you have a place to rest, however negative this perch is. There is a certain satisfaction, a seeming solidity that comes with discovering your "real problem." Now fixing yourself becomes an entirely straightforward proposition: Heal your inner child; rewire your brain; take a medication; relive your trauma; quit sugar; find groups of fellow sufferers to rehash your experiences with. However, you may know from personal experience that none of these approaches will remedy your addiction. Instead, defining yourself as damaged and deciding you are spiritually or physically impaired can reinforce your worst behaviors.

The causes and manifestations of addiction are infinitely complex. Searching for a single cause—and, by extension, a single cure—is simplistic, unnecessary, distracting, and obviously counterproductive. Say, for example, you trust the expert who tells you that your addiction stems from childhood trauma. Of course, there will be evidence to support this explanation because we all have bad memories with which to fill in those blanks. But, what if you cannot recall anything life-altering? What if this explanation doesn't sit right with you? Do you embark on the program anyway, believing that you cannot trust your own mind?

CASE: We met Suzanna in Chapter 2. Suzanna was actually an alcoholism researcher herself, in her late twenties. She was popular, but nonetheless a bit of a loner. She had had boyfriends, but nothing lasting. Moreover, she felt her work unsatisfying—that others determined the direction of the research she worked on, while she carried out the grunt work. This despite her sterling academic record, her reliability, and her desire to make a contribution. Moreover, bad feelings regularly surfaced for her, as a result of which she drank steadily, needing alcohol to feel okay. Suzanna was one of three children. Her home had not been a happy one. She never saw her parents embrace, or really talk kindly or considerately to each other. Then, shockingly, when Suzanna was eight, her mother disappeared from her life.

One day, her mother no longer lived with the family. Her father and an unmarried aunt who moved in with her and her siblings explained that she had to leave for important reasons Suzanna couldn't grasp. Only years later, as a teenager, did Suzanna learn that her mother had gone to live with another man—first in their same city, and then moving some distance away.

Although her mother did contact the children—and even visited with them, taking them shopping and to shows from time to time—Suzanna always understood these were to be short outings. At first, Suzanna would cling to her mother throughout these times together, as though she could make them permanent by never letting her mother out of her grasp. But as a teenager, Suzanna came to have a very jaundiced view of such get-togethers and barely showed any interest in them. Nonetheless, she constantly asked herself, "Why did my mother desert me?" She was torn between feelings of inadequacy about herself and anger at her mother. Her older brother seemed untroubled by such feelings. Her sister, close to her age, was even more devastated by the experience than she was. Years later, her sister died in a drug incident.

Suzanna never felt privileged, protected, prized not only as a child, but also as a student and young professional. Nonetheless, she was independent and capable. She threw herself into her studies, wrapping her life around them, achieving success upon success. In pursuing her academic career, she never allowed another person to become a permanent part of her life. She didn't feel she could trust anyone. After gaining a Ph.D., Suzanna became a post-doctoral researcher in a prestigious alcoholism research program. But she never sought out a senior mentor, and her career stagnated.

Seeking to right her emotional state and thus not to require alcohol as an emotional crutch, Suzanna began attending a group of trauma survivors. The leader of the group, a great believer in physically locating the traumas group members had experienced, provided diagrams of the inescapable ways such events damaged the midbrain and limbic system. Suzanna didn't identify completely with this scenario, because it wasn't necessarily the specific moment her mother left that depressed her, so much as the cumulative experiences of her upbringing and dealings with her parents.

What if we replace "childhood trauma" with "powerlessness" or "impulsiveness" or any number of universal human experiences or characteristics that could just as easily (or not) be the root cause of addiction? The only people who are truly helped by zeroing in on a single problem are the experts, who are sure to touch a nerve and can then build their program on that single premise. That's not to say that these negative elements aren't important and worth your attention. This was critically true in Suzanna's case. There is no denying or ignoring the enormity of losing one's mother or father, particularly when they desert a child and the family.

You may have suffered deeply as a child, with serious emotional effects—even as others who underwent comparable experiences did not or, perhaps, had even worse consequences. These experiences may have searing effects on your life, and you may have done self-destructive things in their wake. But there is a difference between accepting these things as one part of you, on the one hand, and using them to explain and determine the rest of your life, on the other.

CASE: Beth was a successful lawyer who drank heavily at times. As the years went by, she found that she just didn't have the stamina she used to. Hangovers began to interfere with her work and sense of well-being. This feeling that she was not the master of her life was foreign and unsettling to her. She sought help from an expensive, private addiction specialist, an ardent follower of the Adult Children of Alcoholics (ACoA) movement.

During their first session together, the two discussed Beth's childhood, which Beth did not consider particularly traumatic. Her parents loved her. She appreciated them and knew they had done their best. "On the weekends," Beth told her therapist, "Mom and Dad would drink steadily, starting with Manhattans on Friday after work and ending with an all-day Sunday hangover." Indeed, this pattern was fairly common in their upscale social milieu at the time. It may seem odd, but Beth remembered these rituals almost fondly. There had never been incidences of abuse, and

Hangover Sunday was actually a pretty cozy day, with the family lounging around together, having dinner on TV trays in front of *60 Minutes*.

Beth's therapist had a completely different perspective on her memories. Gently, but very assuredly, she pronounced that Beth was not only an alcoholic, but also an Adult Child of Alcoholics. Beth accepted her therapist's assessment, even if it didn't sit right with her. But she assumed that was her resistance operating and wanted to trust the therapist, who was charging her a hefty fee.

Beth quit drinking altogether as the best policy for her. But she maintained deep misgivings about what she was learning. At the same time, she accepted that her mind was warped and would try to deceive her. She was afraid *not* to believe that. Beth began to view everything she had worked for in her life as nothing more than a symptom of child-of-alcoholics pathology. She became almost ashamed of the things that used to bring her pride and a sense of purpose and meaning.

But all this wasn't helping Beth feel any better about herself. She wondered if this proved she was deeply in denial. Out of the blue, she consulted a therapy directory and found Mike. When she entered his office, Beth felt a whole different aura. Mike was cheerful; even his handshake was encouraging—"We're going to do good work together," he enthused.

Almost instantly, Mike strived to get beyond Beth's rehashing whether her parents were alcoholics and she an ACoA. "Let's review all of your accomplishments. Your success at work, and especially your success in rearing your daughter." Beth was married with an adult daughter. Her daughter also had a good career and a sound marriage. Moreover, her daughter was a *moderate* drinker.

Mike's approach was novel for Beth. You mean therapy wasn't about ferreting out your deepest, innermost, never-to-be-resolved problem? "Can you tell me how you were able to help your daughter learn to drink moderately?" Mike questioned Beth. "I drank carefully in front of her . . . You know, I actually asked her that recently. She said, 'Mom, how could I have done anything else when you loved me so much?'"

Let's return to the values assessment you completed in Chapter 4, this time answering only the second half, which focuses on your skills, gifts, and accomplishments.

VALUES QUESTIONNAIRE

6. What key skills or talents do you have?

7. What are your most positive qualities?

8. Name at least two accomplishments or events that you are proud of: Did you help someone? Did you win a competition? Did you build or create something? Did you stand up for something you believe in?

9. Who are the most important people in your life, either people you really care about, or people you can really count on, or both?

10. Which three human values do you elevate most, such as kindness, generosity, friendship, honesty, hard work, creativity, independence, integrity?

Imagine the things Beth might enter in response to this survey: Her brilliance as a lawyer. The skills and thinking that gained her respect. Her professional colleagues. Her family (how *did* she produce a moderate-drinking daughter?). Like Beth, you have successes and accomplishments. You have strong areas of your life, skills, and other assets, including your own values. You're not a blank slate for somebody or something to imprint *their* mark on. Your answers tell you a lot about who you already are. Nonetheless, the function of this exercise is to recognize the as yet unleashed power of your personal resources, ones you have neglected, quarantined, or not given the time and place to develop more fully.

What Is Self-Acceptance?

Self-acceptance is a fundamental concept in contemporary psychology. Think, first, of all the girls who have negative self-images because of how they look at their bodies, of Alexis and other anorexics and bulimics. Self-acceptance is also, in the form of the concept of "loving kindness," a precept of Buddhist philosophy. Self-acceptance and loving kindness are compassion for yourself and the belief that you, like everyone else, are entitled to fulfillment and joy. In her book *Radical Acceptance*, Buddhist psychologist Tara Brach describes the two sides of self-acceptance: "seeing clearly, and holding our experience with compassion." Mindfulness is the essence of seeing clearly. And now we must bring compassion to our clarity. Compassion, as Brach describes, "is our capacity to relate in a tender and sympathetic way to what we perceive," including our vision of ourselves. Self-acceptance is grasping emotionally and intellectually that there is nothing so different or wrong with you that you are disqualified from being a part of humanity and claiming what life offers you. When you address your addiction, you realize that, yes, you have made mistakes; no, your life is not a mistake in the universe.

Put yourself in the position of a parent of a child whose physical features do not meet the cultural ideal. Let's say she has a large nose. Of course, you believe—and strive to make clear to the child—that she or he is not defined by her nose, that she is not disqualified from any activity by her nose, and that kids with less prominent noses all harbor their own individual quirks. One may have an ideal nose, but happen to be carrying some extra weight. Another might have a developmental disability. While yet another might have infinite freckles. The parent is not primarily oriented to noting other children's deficiencies, of course. Instead, she wants to convey to her daughter what a beloved, talented, appealing human being *she* is.

The truth here is that all these children—each of whom falls short of perfection—deserve to participate in a joyous adventure together, no matter what their peculiarities. Perhaps you can see where this is going and can follow this analogy to its logical conclusion for you, as a child of nature. And it is a *logical* conclusion.

Reflection: Self-Compassion

When you view another person through the panoramic lens of compassion—as you would for any child born on this planet—superficial standards of perfection are irrelevant. Compassion is not blindness to negativity. It is perspective. It's the ability to see both flaws and ideals as incidental to the whole, which is abiding. Everyone, including you, deserves to participate fully in life. Your positive qualities don't entitle you to fulfillment, but neither do your negative qualities disqualify you. Surely you, like everyone else, have areas that need attention—areas that hinder you from honoring the things you value. Addiction—among other things—is one significant such hindrance. And these negative attributes of yours can never excuse your not honoring what matters most, or prevent you from doing so. If you feel some resistance to viewing yourself compassionately, remind yourself that this is the most rational and healthy perspective, the way you would treat any child, any young person, any fellow human being. Reread and *think about this*.

Exercise 2: Self-Compassion

Make a list of the negative traits that you believe you are saddled with. Next to each trait, record how it makes you feel to believe this about yourself. (Don't worry—we'll complete Exercise 1, Part 3 shortly!)

- How did you come to believe this about yourself? Did you hear it from someone?
- Now, can you think of a time when you behaved in a way that emphasized the opposite characteristic? For instance, if you listed that you are selfish, remember when you behaved generously and write about that experience. Now, think of another time. How does it make you feel to remember this/these experience/s?
- How realistic is it for you to believe that you are defined by that negative trait? Put that negative quality in a more realistic perspective in terms of your whole life.
- Imagine that you are speaking to a beloved friend with the same negative characteristic. What would you tell him or her if they said they were overwhelmed by their own worst trait?

Self-Acceptance in The PERFECT Program

True recovery is built on self-acceptance, which begins with embracing a view of yourself as someone who deserves a normal, fulfilling life. You cannot start down a path that will lead you toward wellness and peace of mind if you do not believe that the best life has to offer is for you, too. Taking action to overcome addiction is, after all, an act of self-care. So, instead of beginning your journey by looking for something that's wrong with you, let's start by embracing what's already right and then building on that. As well as your deserving the best, the people and things (values, connections, accomplishments) you care about deserve your best.

Exercise 1, Part 3

Revisit your original answers to the question, "I want to recover from addiction because . . ." and your reflections about how negative your view of yourself is. Focusing on negative pronouncements, shift your perspective to one of compassion and objectivity, and see if your earlier statement still makes sense. For instance, maybe you can see that you are not a terrible parent, but a loving parent who has behaved in ways that you would not if you were free of your addiction. In the second column, write down these more realistic observations.

By this point, even if you see that self-acceptance is the rational, healthy approach, it still takes real effort to apply it to yourself. Habits of mind are hard to break, and that's why *self-acceptance, or loving kindness, is a practice*, in exactly the same way that mindfulness is a practice, and not an instant revelation. What's more, self-acceptance is a more challenging practice, because it tends to confront and even activate our fears about ourselves, causing us to respond defensively. For instance, deliberately working to accept the idea that you are not a social misfit can actually feel frivolous and embarrassingly self-indulgent. Imagine how it would feel to repeat the phrase, "I love you, [your name here]," out loud to yourself. Just thinking about this scenario—let alone actually doing it—probably makes you cringe.

Don't worry—I won't ask you to do that one. It's pretty advanced! Instead, the exercises will introduce you to a meditation that has its roots in the Buddhist practice of loving kindness. That is, the deliberate cultivation of compassion, which goes hand-in-hand with mindfulness. Clarity and self-acceptance are the cornerstones of your reclaimed life, ones that you will reinforce in creating new habits of mind. In referencing Buddhist practices here, I am not encouraging you to adopt a religion. (I *will* note that Buddhism does not have a higher-power, God concept, which has led courts to rule that it is unconstitutional to force Buddhist practitioners to participate in AA.)[7] As I've said throughout, this thousands-year-old practice replicates important contemporary psychological and therapeutic concepts. And even the idea of "practice" strongly suggests the modern cognitive-behavioral principle underlying *Recover!*—that you do best and most readily that which you have rehearsed doing until it becomes a natural response for you.

Exercise 1, Part 4

After having listed your reasons for wishing to escape addiction in the first column, then assessing how negative they can be and recasting these in positive ways in column two, now move to the third column and reframe your answers to "I want to overcome addiction because . . . " based on your middle-column revisions. For example, you might replace "I am a terrible parent," with "So I can be present and involved in my children's lives every day." The point of this exercise is to help you internalize the positive, life-affirming reasons for beating your addiction. If you can think of any more ways that living addiction-free will have a positive impact on your world, please list them here, too.

Forgiveness

Addicts are known for excusing all sorts of misdeeds toward others and society. But there appears to be little difference between such shallow notions of self-forgiveness and sociopathy—whatever I do for myself is fine, is justified. So how is it possible for you to "let go" of the guilt you may carry for destroyed relationships, broken promises, deteriorating health—even instances of betrayal and violence? How (like Rose) do you forgive yourself for letting down a child or squandering your dreams? It's quite impossible, if we believe that forgiveness means absolution from responsibility or simply moving on as if nothing had happened. *And, yet, a crucial ingredient of self-acceptance is forgiveness of self and, in an act of sister compassion, forgiveness of others.* Just as mindfulness meditation affects addictive behavior and brain centers, compassion can also be learned.[8]

Forgiveness is both a critical element in and a natural result of self-acceptance. Self-deprecation and guilt for past misconduct do not lead to better behavior, as we saw earlier in relation to relapse after feeling shame. Self-control research has discovered that self-criticism *reduces* self-control. Rather, self-acceptance and forgiveness—especially in the face of stress and failure—*enhance* people's capacity for changing negative behaviors. Consider a study of students who procrastinate, then beat themselves up for having done so. The very act of self-recrimination for procrastinating makes it *more* likely that they will do so again before future exams. *The harder the students were on themselves, the greater this effect.* Thus, "forgiveness, not guilt, increases accountability . . . taking a self-compassionate point of view on a personal failure makes people more likely to take personal responsibility for the failure than when they take a self-critical point of view. They also are more willing to receive feedback and advice from others, and more likely to learn from the experience."[9]

The seeming paradox that being kinder to yourself makes you more ready to accept negative feedback follows from Freudian psychology as well. The energy spent defending your ego—like that used for patchwork on your addicted self—diverts you from the essential changes you need to make. And, so, the opposite of self-forgiveness is as likely to be self-protective defensiveness as it is to be self-abuse. Both end up at the same place—maintaining your self-defeating behavior.

CASE: George and Melissa's child, Sam, was having behavioral problems at school. When presented with his parenting deficiencies, George immediately became defensive: "So, I'm a bad parent!" The only alternatives for George were, first, to blame his own father and mother for their poor parenting; second, unfortunately, to offset the negative feelings he had about his own parenting by labeling Sam with this or that condition to excuse his misbehavior. This then contributed to George's remonstrating and punishing Sam, which sometimes dominated their interactions.

Instead of having the therapy be about saying that he was a bad parent, the family therapist emphasized, they were all in the business of allowing George to interact more constructively with Sam: for instance, by distracting Sam with positive activities when he acted out, by praising him, and by causing him to be mindful (as age-appropriate!) about his acting out. "Sam, I wonder how you were feeling when you hit that boy at school. How did you feel afterwards, and when the teacher sent you home?" As George relaxed within himself over the course of therapy, his self-forgiveness created a chain reaction of his showing greater tolerance for Sam's behavior while Sam in turn became more self-accepting and, as a result, better behaved.

Now let's define the alternative to self-protective defensiveness as forgiveness of a type that reflects compassion and realism. Even if you are not ready or able to completely release the emotional pain, you can strive not to be guilt-ridden. It may feel to you, at this moment, that you don't deserve to live without guilt: You willingly take on the painful burden of self-reproach as penance. That is normal, but I hope you will accept this insight along with your pain: Grasping for pain by ruminating on and reliving your worst moments will keep you stuck in pain—*and pain begets further pain.* Anything you have done to harm or betray yourself or others was done from a place of pain. So, your journey to true recovery is not simply a selfish gift to yourself, but a genuine act of atonement to the family and friends you may have hurt or betrayed. Lifting yourself out of the painful frame of mind and heart that would allow you to perpetuate destructive behavior begins with forgiving yourself.

Reflection: Self-Forgiveness

Forgiveness is not an event. It is a *process* of releasing paralyzing emotional pain by focusing compassionate and understanding attention on your memories and feelings of remorse or grief. Reread and *think about this*.

CASE: Harry abandoned his girlfriend and their young daughter, Anne. He had no interest in family life or the responsibility involved. He tried here and there, but the hit to his freedom made him seethe. He had a regular barstool at the local pub, and it missed him keenly when he was elsewhere. That felt more like home to him than his apartment with his girlfriend and daughter. So, he just dropped out of their lives and became a deadbeat dad—missing child support payments, missing birthdays, going months without a phone call. Sometimes he felt like a heel, when he thought about it. But more often, he cynically used his estrangement from his daughter—blaming it on the girlfriend—to garner sympathy from women at the bar, going on and on, drink in hand, about how he missed Anne, wished he could see her grow up.

Grow up Anne did. And Harry missed it. As a teenager in high school, Anne treated him like a distant relative, which he was. But now, as a middle-aged man with less interest in barstools and barflies, Harry was overwhelmed with regret. There are no do-overs in situations like this. Harry had blown it. His guilt grew into a persistent self-loathing, the pain of which he still alleviated at the bar, albeit during briefer periods spent there. The change was superficial; Harry was still indulging the same behaviors that had brought him to this point. He missed his daughter's graduation—not simply because he'd rather be partying, but because he now felt that he didn't deserve to celebrate her accomplishments with her.

For her part, despite the fact that she was used to his missing her milestones, Anne was nonetheless hopeful that Harry would show himself, and then disappointed when he didn't show, a pattern that never failed to dismay her.

Harry's profound remorse kept him paralyzed, stuck in a life that perpetuated and deepened his own and his daughter's pain. It's true that he can never make up for the lost time and can never undo the damage his abandonment did to his relationship with his daughter, nor can he fix the hurt he had caused. Perhaps he deserves a life of loneliness and regret for the choices that he made. However, wouldn't it be better for everyone whose lives Harry touches if he could influence his social sphere in a positive way? It might be satisfying—to observers and to Harry himself—to know that he is suffering. But as long as he is consumed with self-loathing, he will continue to hurt the people around him, including his daughter.

Shifting perspective to one of compassion for Harry, we can provide a context of understanding for his behavior. Harry had been emotionally abandoned himself as a child. His parents were divorced, his father was a deadbeat dad, and his mother raised Harry along with three other children. So he came into fatherhood having no experience of it as a child or a man, believing that he was incapable and unworthy of it. Now, understanding what happened and why is not the same as absolving Harry of responsibility for his behavior. He has to live with it. What he does have, however, is the opportunity to influence future outcomes: to become a healthy, positive influence on his daughter's life from here on. To do that, he must begin the process of self-forgiveness.

The 12-step practice of "making amends" (step 8) involves going to all of the people you have harmed in your life, acknowledging to them that you have hurt them, and telling them that you're sorry. It sounds like the correct thing to do. However, in AA, amends is an event, like confession, and once you have made your apology, you are absolved and need never revisit your misdeeds. This is in keeping with AA's "keep your own side of the street clean" philosophy and its essentially selfish—"look after yourself"—program. "Amends" plays out the idea that one makes amends for oneself—to support one's own sobriety—not to establish an understanding with the people one has harmed, or even to develop a new aspect of one's own personality, view of life, and actions. Thus, amends-makers are told that it is none of their business whether the recipient of their amends is receptive or not. You've done your job when you apologize.

Granted, you cannot control whether or not others forgive you or choose to reinstate you within their community. But to believe that you have done your part by apologizing and that it is "their problem" if they don't accept your contrition lacks the depth and maturity of genuine compassion and accountability. Harry has apologized to his daughter more times than he can count, and has even felt sorry for himself when his overtures have not resulted in her immediately embracing him and all his faults. For Harry, forgiveness requires an interwoven three-part journey, one that requires him to forgive himself, to seek forgiveness from his daughter, and to forgive his own parents—each part influencing and supporting the others. Let's examine each one separately.

In order to forgive himself, Harry must start by taking a broader view of his behavior, opening with the understanding that he is not, at his core, a selfish, irresponsible, irredeemable human being. He has behaved in ways that he is ashamed of, but the very fact that he can feel shame and remorse indicates that there is a wise heart alive within him, just as your recognition of your flaws and mistakes shows your own wise heart.

Broadening his perspective on his inner landscape to include his wise heart will allow Harry to bring the lenses of compassion and understanding to bear on his interpretation of his past behavior. Where he once saw nothing but coldness, he might now recognize fear. Where he once saw selfishness, he might now see the floundering of an abandoned child. And where he once saw intractable negative qualities, he might now see a path opening into possibility, even redemption. At the point where he can see that transformation through self-forgiveness is possible for him, Harry confronts a straightforward choice, but one difficult to make. He can choose to live in guilty pain, or to release it.

Harry's potential act of self-forgiveness may provide cold comfort to his daughter, and, indeed, she may never forgive him no matter how profound his transformation. Continuing down the path illuminated by his wise heart, regardless of her acknowledgment—respecting her boundaries without expectation and without believing that her rejection or resentment is "her own problem"—is one way Harry can honor the pain he has caused her and genuinely change the situation and the people involved in it. Whether or not his daughter chooses to forgive him, Harry can still live a life infused with compassion and understanding for her, allowing him to cease making decisions that cause her more grief. Even should Anne forgive her father, she might choose to maintain her distance from this virtual stranger, whom she has known to be toxic and who has brought such disappointment. Her own wise heart prevents her from continuing to put herself in harm's way.

Harry may include his own parents on his journey to forgiveness. Again, he has the choice to continue ruminating on the wrongs done to him and the devastating effects they have had on his life, to feel sorry for himself and bitter. Or he can view these things with forgiveness in order to release his own feelings of abandonment. He may be able to see that his mother was tired and overwhelmed when she neglected him—that she simply was not able to be a nurturing caretaker. Perhaps now he might see that she was doing the best she could. Harry can acknowledge the heartache his mother's withholding caused him as a child. But extending compassion to her now allows him to begin down the path of healing as an adult. And being able to see that her behavior was an indictment not of his lovableness, but of her capacity to express love, reinforces Harry's ability to love himself. In other words, Harry's choice to forgive others is bound to his ability to forgive himself, which in turn gives him the ability to seek forgiveness from and make genuine amends to Anne and others he has harmed.

It is a common platitude to say that forgiveness is a gift we give ourselves. The underlying message in that aphorism is that we don't forgive people who harmed us to let them off the hook; we do it so that *we* are off the hook, so that we can move on with life and be better ourselves. While it's true that we forgive for our own well-being, our well-being has an impact on everyone and every situation we come into contact with—past, present, and future. To expand on the notion that it is a gift we give to ourselves, bear in mind that self-forgiveness is essential to true recovery. Releasing your pain of remorse or self-loathing is no easy thing. But doing so is freeing.

Reflection: Harm Reduction and Forgiveness

In Chapter 3, I introduced the concept of harm reduction—the idea of curtailing the addiction script of "in for a penny, in for a dollar." That is, the idea that you've already made a mistake, so why not make it a doozy—if you've had a drink, go all out and expose yourself to the worst dangers possible. We will see the reversal of this script again in the practice of "relapse prevention," in which you pull up short on your incipient bender. The same pattern and its opposite apply to your deteriorating relationship with someone you care about.

Notice how Harry's guilt caused him to continue to turn away from his daughter, exacerbating his alienation from her. This is typical of addictive patterns, where one bad feeling begets others, until your whole attitude cascades into a total abandonment of the situation—and often consciousness—at the cost of further failure and bad feelings. Can you find an example where this has occurred in your life, where your initial overreaction led to bad feelings between you and a loved one that fed off each other? As painful as reimagining such a situation can be, think now how you might have practiced forgiveness at the outset and avoided such bad consequences including, perhaps, the end of the relationship? Think how the other person involved in the situation might have responded differently, more positively, and your life would be richer today.

Perhaps now you are prepared to make forgiveness your practice the next time you face such a situation. Or perhaps you are not quite ready to stop ruminating over something you did or something someone did to you, or beating yourself up over something you may continue to do. In those cases, you can begin planting the seeds of forgiveness by simply allowing for the possibility of release. Be aware of the trap you may set for yourself by heaping more reproach on yourself for your resistance to change. Just like recovery, mindfulness, and self-acceptance, forgiveness—as I said—is a process. If you are struggling with self-forgiveness because you find it difficult to accept the harm you have caused yourself or others, or because others have wounded you in a way that keeps you in a state of heartache, you can start the process of forgiveness—make room for it in your heart—now.

Which brings us back to Suzanna, the twenty-something alcoholic alcoholism researcher. Suzanna, of course, is in a role similar to Anne's or Harry's with respect to their parents. Moreover, she drinks to mask her pain, the pain of abandonment she always felt from a mother who endangered her by her own selfishness and inadequacy, by leaving her to her father—and to fate. That time has gone. Suzanna is an extremely accomplished and talented survivor, and her mother is still alive and active and wants a relationship with her daughter. Yet, in her late seventies, she is not really in a position to fully acknowledge her forgone sins and her role in Suzanna's problems. In fact, she is not that different from the person she was when she left her family, although she is in a different situation now, living alone, having divorced the man she left them for.

Here is how Suzanna thinks:

> "I don't mean to attempt to relinquish personal responsibility for my actions—that's pointless. But I guess there is some comfort in the thought that maybe I'm not actually weaker than other people on a fundamental level, maybe I'm just still trying to overcome a deep pain, and maybe I'm doing okay. I've always had a strong drive towards personal integrity, had a deep desire to be good, and that includes taking care of my body and my mind. I feel deeply ashamed that I have wasted time, energy, and brain cells on a never-ending quest to feel better. But it's not feeling better that I crave, it's feeling okay, like maybe this life is at least a little bit more than a burden to be suffered through.

> "These are the things that plague me when I don't drink. Drinking makes me happy in the short term, yes. But more importantly, I think, is that it has a sustained effect of dulling negative feelings and quelling intrusive thoughts. And in that way it is the best medication that I have found so far—better than antidepressants!—and I don't know if I'll ever really be able to give it up. And I don't mean drinking a healthy amount either."

As to Suzanna's mother:

> "I am not willing to let go of the emotional pain yet. It serves a purpose, just like drinking does. We learn lessons from pain. I can decide to not beat myself up about it, but I refuse to let it go. I know that my previous experiences of hurt cause me to be wary of strong feelings towards other human beings. Only time will convince me that it is really safe to have such feelings. It may take a long time."

Suzanna, like all of us, is a work in progress. So, what should Suzanna do? Remember, the problems we are concerned with are Suzanna's, and not just forgiveness for forgiveness's sake. What will make her whole within herself, allow her to avoid drinking to self-medicate, and enable her to accept and love herself and enter the world of trusting and intimate relationships? As with Harry, for Suzanna, too, the answer may be forgiveness—or at least acceptance.

Jeannette Walls was asked about her mother, whom she described as selfish and neglectful in her powerful memoir, *The Glass Castle* (Scribner, 2005). For years, Walls avoided her mother, even as the older woman was homeless in New York where Walls was a member of the glitterati. Now Walls's mother lives in a separate residence on her farm. Walls says, "So many people ask, 'How could you forgive your mother for the way you were raised?' It's really not forgiveness in my opinion. It's acceptance. She's never going to be the sort of mother who wants to take care of me."[10]

Moving Forward

All of these decisions and efforts—to strive to forgive, to get beyond pain and negativity—are motivated by larger values you hold: to want to love, to be at one with your family, to be at peace, to be free to accomplish larger goals, to be a good person, and to benefit others and humanity. In the following chapter, we will turn our focus to the elements of your life that are most valuable to you—rediscovering meaning and beginning the process of infusing your life with purpose.

Exercises and Meditations

Meditation: Loving kindness

Loving kindness practice is meant to cultivate compassion by making it a familiar state—a habit of mind. It challenges you to direct compassion toward yourself and to extend it to others. Often, one will begin with a template of sorts—a list of wishes you might have for someone you love unconditionally. For instance:

> May ____ be healthy and whole.
> May ____ be safe from danger.
> May ____ be content and at peace.
> May ____ love and be loved.

Now, please consider someone you love without reservation, and in your Personal Journal make your own list of well-wishes for them. Feel free to use the ones we provided, write your own list, or mix and match.

Every day—when you wake up, when you're walking the dog, before your daily meditation—repeat your list of well-wishes, focusing at first on one or more people you love. Normally, one would use one's self as the first object of the loving kindness meditation, but if you have a difficult time conjuring these feelings for yourself, it will help to start with someone for whom you already feel a more spontaneous sense of compassion. This will allow you to become accustomed to holding compassion in your heart. You are going to keep extending these well-wishes, in this order:

1. Someone you love (or all the people you love)
2. Yourself
3. Someone you are neutral about (perhaps someone you see every day, but don't know well)
4. All of humanity
5. Someone you dislike or harbor difficult feelings about (perhaps a bully)

Repeat your list of wishes at least three times for each object of your compassion, then move on to the next. If this is a lot to take on at once, feel free to approach this practice in small steps over time. Take the time you need to feel comfortable doing this—and making it part of your routine—before extending your practice. You might start by directing your wishes only toward your beloved and to yourself. When that begins to feel natural, extend your practice—you should always feel challenged as you push your boundaries.

There are many variations and approaches to loving kindness. You can explore and find others. All have the same kernel—an idea, a spirit, an approach to life to which you have now been introduced, and that you can continue to explore while reading *Recover!*, while embarked on the rest of The PERFECT Program, and throughout your life.

Journal exercise

This is an exercise with three components, paralleling Harry's—and Suzanna's related—path to forgiveness. This is a detailed writing project—one that may be emotionally difficult—so allow yourself ample time to complete it, even if that means working on it over the course of a few days.

Begin by writing down in your PERFECT Journal all of the things about you, or things you have done to yourself, some of which you may still be involved in, that you feel are unforgivable or undeserving of compassion. For instance, have you damaged your health or finances through your involvement with addiction?

Next, write down the things you have done to others, or negative situations you believe you are to blame for (which, again, may still be ongoing) that you feel are unforgivable. For instance, have you behaved neglectfully, carelessly, selfishly? Recklessly or violently?

Finally, write down all of the harmful things that have been done to you by others, things you feel you cannot forgive.

Once you have made your lists, review them with the intention of seeing each of these events as the result of some fear, hurt, incapacity, or void in your life or in someone else's. Even if you have believed that your behavior (or someone else's) was due to your own (or someone else's) fundamentally weak or evil nature, make your best guess about what could have allowed for such behavior. Coming up with a reason does not mean that you must immediately extend forgiveness. Rather, this exercise is broadening your understanding enough to allow for the possibility of forgiveness. It opens the door.

Mindfulness meditation: Forgiveness of others along with oneself

Sit comfortably in your meditation spot and bring to mind an event or a personal characteristic for which you cannot forgive yourself or someone else. Remember it in as much detail as possible, and pay particularly close attention to the feelings the memory arouses in you. Bring your mindful attention to those feelings and the physical sensations they produce. Then name these feelings, both emotional and physical, as precisely as possible. For instance, if you feel shame or hopelessness, call them what they are. If those feelings register physically as restlessness, burning scalp, or weakness, name those sensations as well.

Hold those feelings at the front of your mind—tolerating the discomfort if you can—but, as you hold them, imagine expanding the physical space you occupy and the emotional space around those feelings. For instance, imagine that you have expanded into the space around you by six inches. Allow these feelings to exist as they are, but visualize making more room for them. This may take some practice, but when you are able to do this and to hold that open space, shift your perspective into the neutral space and reexplore these hurtful feelings with a compassionate eye. You can do this meditation focusing on self-forgiveness or forgiveness of another.

Like the loving kindness meditation above, the following is a direct meditation to address forgiveness.

The PERFECT Program version of Buddhist forgiveness practice

> *To those whom I may have caused harm, knowingly or unknowingly, through my thoughts, words, and actions, I ask your forgiveness.*

To those who may have caused me harm, knowingly or unknowingly, through their thoughts, words, and actions, I offer my forgiveness as best I am able.

For any harm I may have caused myself, knowingly or unknowingly, through my thoughts, words, and actions, I offer my forgiveness as best I am able.

CHAPTER 6

Rediscover

Integrity—Finding and following your true self

CHAPTER GOALS

- To develop your focus on your true core values and sense of purpose

Starting by:

- Creating realistic expectations for yourself
- Understanding the flow and change in your ability to follow your purpose
- Putting into play a plan to reconnect with your values

Purpose: Keeping your eye on the prize—escaping addiction—is difficult when you're unclear about why you want to pursue that goal. Addiction blurs and distorts the horizons of your life, preoccupying you with its immediate and superficial gratification, so that your true center has become obscured and confused. Even *after* you loosen your addiction's grip, you may still not be able to hew to your true center. So how do you stay the course to wellness, when you find yourself overwhelmed with endless possibilities and frustrating setbacks? Your task is to sharpen your purpose—your *reason* for quitting and steering forward—one that is personally clear and meaningful to you. In this chapter, you will reconnect with what you value most in life, what brings you joy and fulfillment, and begin the process of transforming those values into clear goals, including especially a non-addicted, fulfilling life.

Don't Change, Become

Why your resolve fails

One of the great mysteries of human nature is that we ever feel tempted to continue in—and often fall back into—behaviors that we *know* make us unhappy. You've probably experienced this phenomenon yourself: You want to quit your addiction and enthusiastically adopt a new lifestyle—you even begin down that path, perhaps proceeding a good distance. You look great, feel great, and even get a little evangelical about it all. You can't believe you ever chose the barroom over the family dinner table, or smoking over breathing, or sugar over whole foods. And then you find at some point that you are right back where you were before you seemingly pulled it together. Why is it so easy to give up something new that makes you feel fantastic and revert to a lifestyle that you know full well will make you miserable? How does this happen?

We have already seen, in Chapter 2, that *addiction makes complete psychological sense. It's a natural human response to unmanageable life circumstances, one through which people mistakenly attempt to find purpose and a sense of well-being.* You gain important "benefits" from the addiction, rewards that sustain the addiction and, for a time, sustain you as well. As I noted:

> Addicted people seek refuge in any powerful, consuming experience that allows them to cope with a life that feels meaningless or out of control—a feeling that is both worsened and relieved by their addiction. The addiction further fills countless hours beyond those eaten up in altered states of consciousness or compulsions. Think of all the mental and emotional energy an addiction wastes: days planned around purchasing and consuming the substance or practicing the activity; fielding negative fallout (like angry co-workers, family members, and friends; mounting bills; health problems); making solemn promises to stop; remorse and guilt. Yet, as painful and self-defeating as these feelings are, their predictability sustains addicts and even lends a bizarre sense of purpose to their lives.

So, freeing yourself from an addiction takes some effort. Obviously, keeping off drugs or alcohol or away from another addiction involves something akin to willpower. Recently, researchers and human potential writers have reinvigorated the concept.[1] Experimental psychologist Roy Baumeister found both that willpower can be practiced and exercised (for example, by standing straight, not buying Doritos, and solving difficult puzzles) and that it can be exhausted by overuse (students forced to use willpower in order to resist a snack when hungry, track a boring display, or control their emotions during a tear-jerking movie immediately afterward showed less self-control). All of this is a bit like you might expect, were it not for intervening messages you have received, like the 12-step doctrine ridiculing and dismissing willpower as a tool in recovery.

Baumeister's findings don't add up to easy answers for the withdrawing or sober addict. They suggest both that exercising willpower in many areas enhances your resistance to your addiction and that, having freshly quit an addiction, your willpower is being strained and shouldn't be taxed. Indeed, conceiving that you are exercising willpower (as in dieting or thinking that you can never use a substance again) can actually weaken your resistance. The PERFECT Program reframes self-control so that you see yourself as becoming, rather than as resisting temptation or even as changing. For example, you can view quitting smoking not in terms of overcoming your addiction, but as embracing and perfecting your true core self. Used in this way, willpower research informs my recommendations throughout *Recover!*.

These issues—what can be called motivation—appear in all phases in releasing an addiction, as we shall see both in regard to initial quitting and later in avoiding relapse. To begin, there may be a certain element of disillusionment that accompanies positive life changes. Consider, for example, the longtime restaurant server who opens her own restaurant, after years of fantasizing about being her own boss. She dreams of independence, success, but mostly of serving uniquely delicious food to a packed house of satisfied customers. She has a solid background in food service, has done all the research, and feels that she is ready for, and realistic about, the incredible amount of work it will entail. She dives in, head first. But, after the initial burst of excitement wears off, this new venture becomes her real life. The twelve-hour days become a routine: bookkeeping, managing her staff, fixing appliances. . . . It's no longer a thrill to see the distributors show up to stock the kitchen—those are costly items she must use up quickly by inducing customers to consume them.

There's a bit of a catch-22 in play here, because if she had factored waning enthusiasm and drudgery into her bright plans for the future, she might never have mustered the enthusiasm and energy required to get the ball rolling. But, then, she's not as prepared for the inevitable reality that work is still work, and she is still herself—only now, her responsibilities are more serious and there is more at stake. It is at this point that keeping focused on her sense of purpose is vital. This new restaurant owner can face a crossroads. Feeling overworked and out of her depth could discourage her, causing her to throw in the towel literally, by closing her doors, or figuratively, by carrying on resentfully and martyring herself to her business as it fails. Or, with her eye on the values that inspired her in the first place (independence, creativity, passion for food, love of people)—she could see the drudgery as one element of the big picture that motivates her to succeed.

Overcoming addiction is similar. You may have fantasies about who you would be and what life would be like if you were not held back by your addiction. Those fantasies can give you the inspiration you need to get started, which is a good thing. But, ultimately, you are going to need a reason to keep pursuing your goal when it becomes clear to you that straightening up will not result in instant realization of all your dreams. Here is another restaurant analogy for you: People who are learning to carry trays of food and drinks to tables are taught to keep their head up and their eyes forward, focused on the direction in which they are going. If they look at their feet or at the tray they are carrying, they are prone to lose their balance, and food and drink will inevitably start sloshing around, perhaps hitting the floor. When you embark down the path toward wellness—freedom from addiction—you must employ a similar technique: Keep your focus on your goal. This is easy enough to do when you're carrying a tray full of drinks and you know where you're going with it. It can be much more difficult when you're headed down an unfamiliar, metaphorical path with no clear goal in sight—perhaps some vague destination called *recovery* or *spiritual enlightenment*—which is how you may feel now.

Exercise 1, Part 1

In your Personal Journal, indulge your fantasies. Write down everything you imagine you would be, or would do, were it not for your addiction. Relationships, work, travel, home life, wellness—the whole shebang!

When you're in the thick of addiction, it's easy to conjure up fantasies of the person you could be, in the same way that it's easy to see only booming success and personal satisfaction before embarking on a new business venture. As I said, these fantasies can be very useful and motivating, but they are not sustainable. Not only that, but—as usual—addiction can bring even more confounding obstacles to this common scenario, aside from disillusionment.

CASE: Graham is a plumber, an independent contractor with a spotty reputation. He has a big and charming personality and does solid, high-end work. That is, when he's on his game. But, he's a binge drinker. His weekend benders have become legendary around town, and, although people think he's a great guy who gets the job done right—and even on schedule—he has been losing contracts because customers are wary of hiring him. Graham has never been just a social drinker, a scotch-with-friends or wine-with-dinner kind of guy. Once he starts drinking, the switch is flipped: His sound judgment is replaced with an insatiable appetite for more. *He knows this about himself.*

Despite the single-minded self-obliteration he indulges in, and its resulting blistering, days-long hangover, Graham still manages to stop partying when he has a job to get to. He pulls himself together, full of excruciating regret, believing in his heart that now he will quit for good and all. He never, ever wants to put himself through this again. He also has a family: a wife and two kids. He may not miss work, but he has missed family weekends and date-nights with his wife, among other wholesome personal obligations. So, how is it that, after a couple of weeks or even months off the sauce, when he's feeling good, physically and mentally, Graham is able to talk himself into that "one drink" he knows will lead to another lost weekend? How does he convince himself that enjoying a drink after work will not go the way it always goes? This is a man who never in his life has had the experience of enjoying a single drink—what disconnect from reality allows him to believe he ever will? Why does Graham make such an irrational decision, given his reality, after he has been sober for a period of time? Shouldn't he be stronger and sharper—better able to stand up to temptations—when he escapes the gravitational force of his addiction?

Why is it so easy for some people to change for just a short time, then go off the wagon and give in to temptation? Put more positively, what is the secret to making changes stick? If you have quit an addiction in the past, and wondered how on earth you could ever have lived so self-destructively, only to find yourself right back in the thick of addiction, then Graham's story should ring a bell for you. It is a common experience, and it is baffling. Quitting an addiction can be almost like waking up from a vivid nightmare: The memory of a horrible dream might linger for days, the same way the pain of a particularly brutal hangover or the sting of a mortifyingly shameful episode might linger for a time. The sharp memories of the aftermath of addiction might keep you determined to stay on the wagon. But the immediacy of those memories begins to fade, the same way a nightmare does, leaving you with hazy impressions of what it was really like ("It wasn't *that* bad, was it?—sort of fun, really—none of these daily concerns and worries.").

In other words, focusing on the horrible downsides of the past might *in the short term* start you on the recovery path, as it does episodically for Graham. When you're keenly aware of the misery you are avoiding by quitting your addiction, it is easier to combat challenges to your resolve with the fear of reliving those horrible feelings. This may tie in with the stage you are at in leaving your addiction, as we will see. But, as the memories fade—as they will do—you will have to find other, more sustaining goals and motivations.

Reflection: Self-Forgiveness Versus Self-Excusing

We spent some time in the last chapter talking about forgiving yourself. Keep in mind that ignoring or dismissing the pain you have inflicted on yourself is not the same thing as self-forgiveness. Self-forgiveness springs from mindfulness—or clarity of perception—while forgetting springs from mental sloth, or obliviousness. Self-forgiveness doesn't say, "Oh, that wasn't so bad," when it really was. It says, "That was bad, but it does not define me." Can you reconcile recognizing the negatives of what you have done, sometimes the horror of it, with respecting and loving yourself? Review the answers you gave in Exercise 2 (page 118) and in Exercise 1, Part 4 (page 120), in Chapter 5.

Remember that addiction is a consuming, destructive involvement that captures your time, your mental and emotional energy, your focus. So much of your life as an addicted person revolves around indulging in and recovering from addiction—interspersed perhaps with fantasies of your non-addicted life. But the dreams of who you could be without addiction fade as quickly as do the nightmare visions of the past. In the stark daylight, you find yourself feeling lost in the world, not knowing how to fill your time, even feeling that you don't know who you are anymore without your addiction. Everything does not automatically fall into place once you clean up—in fact, your responsibilities, your burdens, increase. As Rose (in Chapter 1) found, the first realization upon quitting is a recognition of the many neglected things you *must* do—family obligations, work and school, healthy behaviors—along with avoiding your addiction. Like the new business owner, you now have to cope with the challenges of everyday life, and you have to do it without an escape hatch. Like Graham, who believed he could have one drink (while knowing he wouldn't), you might fantasize about taking a quick respite from your addiction. But, for you, early in recovery, this may be a quick respite that doesn't exist.

Finding your true self

It may be helpful to think about this seemingly inexplicable but universal experience of reverting to self-destructive behavior this way: You simply cannot carry out a charade for very long. One-size-fits-all programs that promise quick—but superficial—transformations or spiritual awakenings are impossible for most people to maintain very long, let alone over a lifetime. For you to succeed in recovering from your addiction, you instead want to make meaningful changes that bring your behavior into harmony with what's truly important to you—not by transforming who you are, but by *becoming* who you are, or who you want to be. As a result you grow into your sense of purpose in life, or your true self.

Exercise 1, Part 2

Follow through on those indulged fantasies about who you could be and what you could accomplish once you are free of your addiction. Imagine that these fantasies are reality, and consider what such a life—in all of its corners—would look and feel like. How would you spend your time? Who would you be with? What activities and people would be forever gone—or at least kept at a distance? What feelings—good and bad—would you need to leave behind? What will make you happy, keep you content? Flesh out fully this vision of your future self.

What do you think of it? Are you ready for it?

When memories and dreams fade, and when disillusionment sets in, what you're left with is just you. Who you are. What will satisfy you and bring meaning to your life?

CASE: Rodney is a good-looking and talented young man. He is technically skilled and maintains a good-paying computer job. He also is perpetually stoned on marijuana and flits in and out of relationships, often going from one woman to another on successive weekends.

When he is with each woman, he pays attention to her needs. He is concerned, and the woman feels cared for. But just as quickly, Rodney disappears, often not to surface again for a month or more. If she tries to reach him, Rodney doesn't even answer his cell phone.

One of Rodney's girlfriends moved in with him at one point. He generally came home from work, went into the bedroom, and got stoned. They might eat dinner together, but gradually, as the woman saw Rodney's mind was elsewhere, she moved on to some other activity—reading, watching TV, going out with a girlfriend. Eventually, she moved on entirely.

Rodney is also part of a close-knit nuclear family. His parents have been married for a long time. His sister, like Rodney, has nerdy technical skills. But she settled down young, with a man who was probably her first lover, and had two children—taking an extended leave of absence from her job during her kids' early years.

When Rodney looks at his sister's life, he both envies and rejects it for himself. He wants children himself and often plays with his niece and nephew. Yet he can never imagine actually living his sister's life. He wonders if his brother-in-law really is satisfied, even as he is sure his parents are with their long marriage.

There are two possibilities for Rodney. The first is that his habitual lifestyle is the best expression of who he is. Not everyone is made for family life, and more and more people live alone. We shouldn't assume that settling down should be everyone's ultimate goal in life and that doing so will bring fulfillment. What brings Rodney satisfaction may be his freedom. Perhaps he is conflicted because he feels he should want the benefits of a stable family life and can see how they make other people happy, but he doesn't want them for himself. He might just be another completely self-oriented person—now often termed "narcissistic"—who never really connects with another person.

But, in fact, this turned out not to be true for Rodney.

RODNEY did find someone with whom he wanted to live, Alyssa, who accepted him as he was while encouraging him to advance in his career. Whereas previously he had been content to jog along and maintain his footloose lifestyle, Rodney applied to return to graduate school in information technology.

But Rodney was still not his family's—nor perhaps anyone else's—model of a settled person. Six months into his relationship with Alyssa, Rodney had to move to another city in order to attend the program that accepted him.

Rodney regularly texted and spoke with Alyssa. But he didn't return her expressions of longing to be together. As he put it, "I haven't had any 'withdrawal' from Alyssa. Often my girlfriends—including Alyssa—think I am kind of cold because I don't miss them. I just don't yearn to see them if I know we will see each other in a month or two. That's fine for me.

"I do enjoy living with Alyssa, but I like living by myself also. However, I know I'm more directed and use my time much more efficiently—and smoke a lot less pot—with Alyssa around!"

Rodney has seen and pursued a different option for himself, one that holds out the promise of really fulfilling himself and growing up even though he remains outside of the traditional lifestyle. Whether this means that he will remain permanently off the standard marital and family grid can't be judged as yet—along with what his ultimate use of marijuana will be. But he is nonetheless exploring the realm of true recovery.

Reflection: To Accept, To Change, To Wait

Many people—in some ways everyone—face Rodney's two possibilities. One is to accept some things about himself as probably permanently different from most other people, but not bad or unworthy on that account, and to carve out a different path for himself. The other is to accept himself as he is at the present time: "This is what I am now, and that's okay, but I may not always be this way." You may not be able to determine this about yourself right now. Think about your lifestyle, how you live, in addition to and beyond what may be your addiction. Name three things about it you would most like to change. Do you really want to change them? Do you predict that you will change them? Why will you or might you not?

Stages of Change

Graham and Rodney are people in different stages relative to their purposes in life, and to their substance dependence. Rodney has begun making changes—but he's still figuring out who he's supposed to be. Graham has decided he wants to change in line with an idea he has about who he is, a professional and family man, but he can't stay the course. They are at two different places in relation to their life purposes, or true selves.

You may have heard of a model called "Stages of Change,"[2] which proposes that people who are in the process of quitting an addiction—or we might also say are transforming their lives or finding and following their true selves—follow a certain path, as shown in Figure 6.1.

FIGURE 6.1

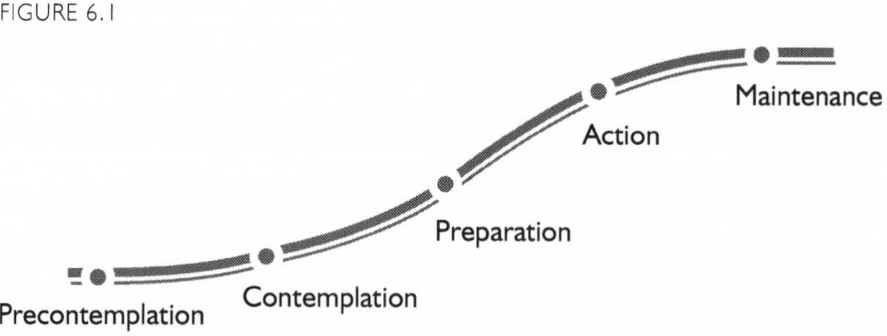

The Precontemplation stage represents a phase in which people are just beginning to tune into their impulse to make a change, but do not yet feel that it is possible. Contemplation is the phase in which change seems like a definite possibility. The Preparation stage is when people are beginning to make plans. And Action is when the plans begin to take effect. Maintenance is the phase where you focus on staying on track. People find this model helpful, in that many do experience some of these phases, and it is perhaps the most referenced addiction change tool.

But I take issue with it in some ways, since the proposed trajectory does not represent a universal reality. Many people's actual experience differs, as common sense and research tell us. People simply do not as a rule follow this exact pattern—they skip steps, reverse direction, spend years in one stage and moments in another. There is no single path to change. Furthermore, the Stages Model does not take into account that the natural maturation process changes people's priorities. Consider Graham's case, for instance: He jumps back and forth between "contemplation" and "action" a couple of times every month. Or, consider Rodney, who was—and to some degree remains in—a prolonged state of precontemplation. Can a person be permanently precontemplative, at least for the majority of their adult life, or are they likely to move beyond that stage? All such possibilities and permutations occur. And, often, when people contemplate parenthood—or become parents—they leap through many stages in a single bound!

The Stages Model can be useful to you, however, if you put a more holistic spin on it by focusing on your identity and true self. Understand that change is not a step-by-step process and that you may experience one or more of these phases at any given time. Furthermore, different areas of your life may go through different stages, just as Graham is mature at work and poorly evolved in his family life. Instead of looking at these stages as a progression that you should pass through in order, look at them as representing different facets of transformation, which do not exist on a hierarchy, but work more like a gyroscope that is continually revolving, sometimes seemingly up, other times seemingly down.

Perhaps the model loses its usefulness if we take away its forward trajectory. What's the point of recognizing these phases if we can't pinpoint where we are on the path, or if we can't use it to get a handle on our progress and look forward to the next step? On the contrary, we can find information and insight that are all the more useful when we apply the model in this real-life way. Let's translate each of the stages into what it means for finding your life purpose, the theme of this chapter, using Rose's story as an illustration. Envision yourself proceeding through each phase yourself, and what that might really look like, in what order and with what timing. Of course, this is just rumination, and your actual experience when embarked on your recovery path may be quite different and may shift as you go along.

Precontemplation: The sense that something is not right. Something doesn't jibe with your principles. But, in terms of purpose, you have not yet solidified what your primary goals are (see Rodney), where you want to be—or head towards—in life. Remember when Rose had first turned to meth and sent her daughter to live with her mother? Of course, she knew something wasn't right. But what, and what to do about it? "Rose's regret loomed in the background. She wished for a do-over; she promised herself that she was going to stop as soon as she finished the drugs she had on hand. Or next week."

Contemplation: You have acknowledged that something is not right and must be changed—but you're not sure how you can realign your life. Here, you may identify important values and a purpose, but you can't yet see how to proceed toward these. Rose, recall, had an epiphany: "Missing her daughter's birthday party had a special impact for Rose, and her thoughts constantly returned to it. It made clear to Rose, as nothing else could, that the costs of her drug use outweighed any benefits that remained from it—even as this would have been obvious all along to anyone with an outside perspective."

Preparation: You now identify how you can bring your values into alignment with your behavior and imagine what these initial steps will be. Rose had to get off a powerful drug, deal with her withdrawal, and reconnect with her real, meaningful life. "When Rose felt that the worst of it (coming off meth) had passed, she called her mother. . . . Her mom came over with a homemade meal. Together they came up with a plan for Rose to reestablish her life, placing what was important at its center."

Action: Taking action, both in the narrow sense of quitting your addiction and in the larger sense of advancing your life—like going to school, dealing with psychological issues, taking control of critical parts of your life. As Rose did:

> With what she was struggling to achieve firmly reestablished in her mind, Rose moved back into her parents' house, rejoining her daughter's daily life. Rose returned to school and found a part-time job at a dentist's office (which was good, because she required considerable dental work). Although she had given up quite a bit of freedom, Rose now shared child-care responsibilities while living with her parents, and that support took enough of the burden off her that she could pursue her studies while sustaining her recovery from addiction.

We turn to your taking these steps in the next chapter.

Maintenance: In PERFECT, maintenance is living a value-driven life, one where you constantly steer according to your purpose and goals, while using relapse-prevention techniques that keep your goals in focus—which I turn to in succeeding chapters. Once again, for Rose:

> Most important was that Rose was able to see the positive results of her changed life and to savor being clean. She was living in harmony with the goals that had been eluding her even before she became addicted. Rose was able to fit both play and quality time with her child into her schedule, as well as spending time with her family. Given where she was coming from, the situation seemed like a dream come true. Beyond this, Rose made space to run and do yoga. Her new circumstances honored the vision she had been working so hard for before her addiction. Now every facet of her life reflected her heart and brought her sense of purpose into sharper focus. She was using her values as a guide to create a place in the world for herself that she had dreamed of.

CASE: Sarah was an investment banker. Although tremendously successful academically and professionally, she was bad at relationships. Instead, she would have periodic alcohol- and drug-fueled intense interactions with men—sometimes lasting a weekend, sometimes a few months.

In her early thirties, Sarah became involved with a man who was far less successful than she was. Of course, that wasn't uncommon for Sarah, and Ron was reliable and capable—he ran the shipping department of a large company.

Ron admired Sarah tremendously and promised her a lifetime of devotion and emotional support. Tired and worried about remaining alone forever, Sarah accepted Ron's suggestion that they marry, and they lived together contentedly, even if Sarah felt the absence of true passion that she had once dreamed of (an experience she shares with many, if you recall the discussion of sex addiction in Chapter 2).

Sarah traveled for her job. During these trips, she began returning to her substance-stimulated affairs. Sarah felt guilty about these and worried that she might be addicted to sex and alcohol. On the other hand, she always returned home to Ron. Indeed, she realized that maintaining her marriage was necessary for her to keep a steady course as an elite financial professional.

Once, as Sarah was considering these things, she was asked to write her bio for a company brochure. As she did so, she recalled how much her work meant to her and how directed she had been in pursuing such a position, a direction she wished ardently to continue. In fact, writing her bio was a values-and-purpose exercise, one that clarified what really motivated her.

By returning to the home base of her true purpose—that of a high-level, skilled, and motivated financial professional—Sarah was able to correct course, both eliminating her affairs and cutting back her drinking (which she had often used as a way to facilitate her sexual interactions). She had assessed her purpose, her true self, and concluded that these steps were a matter of fulfilling her destiny. Of course, Rose made a very similar choice, or refocusing, which neither Rodney nor Graham has yet done. Compared with Sarah, Rose had gone much farther in the course of her addiction, suffering far worse consequences. Would both Rose and Sarah be expected go through the same stages of change, then? They both navigated their true selves in a way that worked for each of them. The method each used wasn't chiseled in stone and delivered to them by God or psychiatry, just as it isn't true that they both went through the same stages of change—or really *any* stages, other than leaving addiction behind. But their successful resolutions were for both a matter of focusing on what was most meaningful in their lives and sticking to that direction and purpose.

Your Values Assessment

In Chapter 3 you filled out your "Values Questionnaire." You returned to it in Chapter 5. The second time you filled it out to assess and appreciate your skills and resources, focusing on the last five items. This time, refocus on the first five and the last two items to locate your true self and purpose.

VALUES QUESTIONNAIRE

1. Name three things that are important to you, whether or not you are actively honoring them right now.
2. What activities would you be pursuing if you were not so occupied with your addiction?
3. Have you abandoned any dreams because of your addiction? If so, name these.
4. What are some things you value that you could lose in the future due to your addiction?
5. What do you hold close to your heart that most opposes your addiction (religious faith, parenthood, political activism, health, self-respect, regard for others, etc.)?

. . .

9. Who are the most important people in your life, people you really care about, or people you can really count on, or both?

10 Which three human values do you elevate most, such as kindness, generosity, friendship, honesty, hard work, creativity, independence, integrity?

Herein, you will find the signposts to your true self. These are the key elements of your life that you may have been ignoring or giving short shrift. The longer you have been living with addiction, the more overwhelmed you may feel by looking at your answers. Let's tackle this list the way a professional organizer or productivity expert would approach a chaotic household or office. You're going to process and sort through your underlying values, what you ultimately care most about, so that you can begin the process of setting goals for yourself that are meaningful to you, that will give your journey a sense of true purpose. This endeavor is like sorting a pile of papers that has accumulated on your desk to the point where you have no place to work, or like cleaning a kitchen that is so out of control that the only appliance you use is your microwave. To accomplish this task, you need a plan of attack.

Organization and efficiency experts will tell you that every stray, homeless item contributes to the chaos in your household and in your life. Anything you see that isn't where it should be or reminds you of something you're supposed to do saps your energy, whether you know it or not. Every unpaid bill, moldy Tupperware container, or unframed picture is like a person staring at you, hoping you'll make eye contact. These things are not accidental, but they are also not necessarily essential to your life. Wherever they fall in your life hierarchy, they *still* represent unkept promises or contribute to a chaotic living situation for you and your family. And they represent a lack of attention to your values. If inanimate objects can have this kind of power, imagine the weight you are bearing under the imploring stare of the values and purpose that are most precious to you, but that you are ignoring.

When you are approaching the daunting task of organizing a physical space full of stuff, you begin by handling each item with the intention of making a few decisions about it: Do you keep it or toss it? Does it need immediate attention? Can it be put off? Is it sentimental? Where does it belong? If you are working with an organization expert, he or she will withhold judgment about what is of value to you. That is up to you to determine. You are going to follow the same principle here, using your answers from your values questionnaire. Reviewing your list might inspire some self-recrimination or feelings of shame for time or dreams lost. If so, summon your foundational mindfulness and self-acceptance practices to guide you here. Like the professional organizer, do not judge yourself; rather, focus on holding yourself and your difficult feelings with mindfulness and compassion.

Exercise: Sorting Your Values

In your PERFECT Journal, process each of your answers to the Values Questionnaire, 1–5, 9 and 10, into one of the following categories—it's okay if they overlap. And feel free to add your own categories.

Things that bring you joy:

Things you believe in:

People you cherish:

Dreams and goals:

Strengths and positive qualities you possess:

This exercise shows you that you do have a true north. These categories represent the important areas of your life—your values—where you will find inspiration, meaning, and purpose. These are your reasons for pursuing freedom from addiction. Feel free to add more items to your list. You can place it where you will see it regularly, like over your desk or by your bed.

Moving Forward

To find the values and purpose that allow you to take—and keep—an addiction out of your life, you need to explore what's important to you and sort through competing demands. In the next chapter, you will begin mapping your way toward actualizing your visions for the future—making your visions real through concrete plans and actions.

Further Exercises

Personal Journal

Carve out some private time before bed, every evening, and review how you spent your day. In your Personal Journal, identify the things you did and the choices you made that reflect your values. For instance, if you decided to cook a healthy dinner instead of ordering take-out or if you did a favor for a friend, record that event and make note of what personal value or values you supported. You might be able to name just one, or more than one.

Exercise

Make a date with yourself and put it on your calendar when you do the values exercise, or as soon as you can after you have done your basic sorting. On that date review your list of values and list one activity you have undertaken in that interim that honors each value. Perhaps you made time to watch a movie you have always loved or spent time alone on another favorite activity, did a favor for a friend, read up on something you have been wanting to pursue, planted some flowers . . . you know the things you value and consider important. Write about how you feel about those things you've done. Make special note of any values not pursued in this time, and list those values for the next review date you set going forward.

Meditation

Envision a time when you have been fully engaged in an activity that has nothing to do with your addiction. You might have to think back to childhood, when imaginative games could feel so important, satisfying, and creative. It might be when you play a sport. Or when you swim at the beach. Or when you see a scary or adventure movie. Do your best to remember what it has felt like to be so fully engaged in something that you don't have to think about what it is that you want; you are just doing it. Bring your mindfulness skills to this meditation and focus on the sensations you experience when remembering this time: What feelings does this memory conjure up? Does it recall certain smells or textures or vistas or people? Do you actually feel different *physically*? Spend as much time as you can exploring in your mind—occupying—this event.

CHAPTER 7

Fortify

Coping—Learning the skills for life management

CHAPTER GOALS

- To assess your strengths and weaknesses
- To implement new life skills
- To discover resources for effective living
- To address mental health issues

Purpose: This chapter focuses on the essential skills and practices that will help you navigate the world freely, non-addictively, and effectively. These are broad subjects, each touched on in a variety of ways. They include practical ideas about skills that will enable you to connect to the world—such as listening, anger management, accepting others, and decision making—combined with brief introductions to cognitive-behavioral techniques such as social network therapy, reciprocity marital counseling, problem solving, assertiveness, the community reinforcement approach (CRA) and family training (CRAFT), and motivational interviewing. You will also contemplate setting and respecting boundaries—your own and others'—and consider the crucial question of boundaries in therapy, and especially in addiction treatment.

Living with addiction, every day you encounter the same scenarios, navigate the same problems, meet the same demands—all centered around your addiction. By remaining focused on this infinite loop of addiction, you neglect important areas of your life. Your home, family life, or finances may be in disarray. You may not know how to cope maturely with stressful situations, hiding in addictive behaviors rather than facing and handling whatever life throws your way. Freedom from addiction allows you to embark on life's adventure, a forward path with goals to set and meet. But living out your true self requires coping skills that you failed to develop on your circular path, making it difficult for you to handle the twists and turns—and sometimes tedium—present in even the most productive and fruitful lives. This chapter is dedicated to providing you with resources and tools for effective living.

Defining "Life Skills"

Do you know people who seem to manage their lives with uncanny effectiveness? They're able to meet the demands of family life, work, and community, and still have time for leisure activities. They don't seem burdened by endless problems that defeat their goals and happiness. In fact, they have learned how to prioritize and to concentrate: to determine what's important and to navigate a path through life focusing on activities in a way that reflects what is most meaningful to them. These highly effective people at the same time deal with stress—conflicting demands, family and personal dynamics, unexpected problems, and even trauma. They aren't people without troubles. They are people who keep these problems in perspective and deal with them without losing track of their larger goals.

In the previous chapter, you took the initial step toward effective living by establishing your priorities—determining what is of ultimate value to you—and setting your course. Now, you will turn your attention toward developing the practical skills you need to follow the course you set for yourself. People may acquire these skills as a matter of course on their way to adulthood. The myopia and all-consuming nature of addiction, however, can hinder you in these key areas, even bring you to a complete halt, making the demands of everyday living seem overwhelming and unmanageable.

If you have always coped with stressful situations by getting high or running outside to smoke a cigarette or stomping out of the house to get drunk, how will you respond to stress once your addictive behavior is off the table? If you have allowed yourself to go into deep debt and have dealt with creditors by refusing to answer the phone and letting the mail pile up unopened while you continue, single-mindedly, looping around your circular addiction path, what do you do about your financial improvidence now that you can see clearly? Do you know how to budget? Or, say you dream of going back to school, but when you start to do the research, you find yourself stymied by all the requirements and options. How do you pursue this goal effectively?

The range of life skills that allow you to live up to the standards of your priorities is very broad, and you may not need help in every area that I am going to cover in this chapter, which is like a crash course in adulthood. One abiding truth about the nature of recovery from addiction is that a large majority of people who experience addiction will "mature out" of it. Many do this on their own, through the natural process of shifting priorities that goes hand in hand with growing up. But, for others, who find themselves blinking into the light after years of addiction, it doesn't come quite so naturally. And the thing they most lack for completing this process is the skills required for coping. These skills cover a lot of ground, so let's break them down into categories.

- Anti-addiction skills
- Decision making
- Goal setting
- Coping skills
- Communication skills: Listening
- Emotional skills
- Boundary setting
- Boundaries and addiction treatment
- Effective therapies: CRAFT and motivational interviewing

Each of these categories encompasses a dense set of subcategories—a chapter could be devoted to each one. And, indeed, in my previous books—like *The Truth About Addiction and Recovery* and *7 Tools to Beat Addiction*—I have put together whole sections of detailed coping skills (like problem solving, anger management, communications, etc.). These have been developed by psychologists who have observed closely the deficiencies that people with addictions often display. I won't be repeating—but only alluding to—these in *Recover!*. The information in this chapter will provide guidelines in these areas, and you can find more detailed descriptions of each as needed in my earlier works.

People can develop severe, life-disturbing problems in any—or all—of these areas. And no one of them stands out as causing addiction. Not everyone will need support with every skill. For instance, you may be very high functioning despite your addiction and need help with only a few. Or, you may need guidance in all of them. With that in mind, I will offer an exploration of these categories and provide you with exercises, resources, and direction so that you can continue your development in the areas with which you feel you need the most help. In fact, discovering and using resources is an important life skill itself. In reading this, you are already beginning to practice that critical skill.

Anti-Addiction Skills

Recover! is all about overcoming addiction, so an anti-addiction section might seem redundant. Following The PERFECT Program, you are approaching your addiction holistically—from all areas of your life. You are realizing a new overall perspective and establishing a completely different foundation for living. But, in doing so, you will face daily challenges to your resolve and will struggle with addictive compulsions and urges. Anti-addiction skills are those practical, systematic ways of dealing with these addictive urges before—or as soon as—they arise.

Addicted people have different triggers—situations that instigate a pull toward destructive behaviors. These might include stress, boredom, depression, just plain habit (like grabbing a cigarette when you're talking on the phone or a bag of potato chips when your favorite TV program is on), or returning to a familiar environment where, or seeing people with whom, you previously engaged in your addiction. Oddly, it is also common—as Alan Marlatt and his colleagues indicate in *Relapse Prevention*[1]—for people to be drawn back to addictions when they are feeling elated or triumphant. As one young female alcoholic athlete described her drinking career: "When was I driven to drink? Whenever we had a big victory, I celebrated. Oh, of course, whenever we suffered a tough loss, I drank to drown my disappointment and depression." And, as I discussed in the last chapter, the tendency to relapse may even occur for some when they are most positive and confident about their recovery.

Sometimes, a gentle urge to get high or binge will present itself seemingly out of the blue. You may dismiss it, but find that what started as an innocuous, stray thought morphs for you into inevitability. Let's explore some of these scenarios and practical ways of dealing with them.

Exercise: Addictive Triggers

What are your addictive triggers? For some, simply waking up in the morning is enough: you might open your eyes and reach for your pack of cigarettes or for your computer to check in on your online game, or obsess over whether your last date or hoped-for love has e-mailed you. Or maybe it's at night when you have finished with your work schedule or other daily obligations. It could also be a place you pass or find yourself in, like a bar, or a group of people—like those you usually drink or get high with. Or it could be a mood—such as boredom or stress or anxiety—that compels you to go to the refrigerator or out for a snack.

When are your cravings the strongest? If you are not sure what triggers you, spend a week keeping track in your PERFECT Journal on a page earmarked "triggers." Make note of the time of day when addictive urges are strongest, what you are doing at the time, what your mood is, and whether or not you are able to overcome them each time.

Have a plan in place

When a craving arises, or when you anticipate that an urge will arise in a certain situation, be prepared for it. Have a few ideas for activities you can engage in when cravings or urges appear, relying on the things that are important to you. Make a list, both in your Journal and to be kept handy, because you may not be able to recall these things when you're in the throes of a desire to indulge. These could be short-term—but enjoyable or satisfying—distractions, like taking a walk, playing catch or doing some other activity with your child, composing an e-mail, weeding a garden, calling your mother or a friend. If you are headed someplace where you know you may face triggering opportunities, have other destinations available to which you can divert your path—the library, grocery store, a coffee-only café, a friend's house, the gym.

Other times, you will be triggered by your daily routines. If, for instance, your usual habit has been to get high as soon as you come home from work, simply walking in the door will be a powerful trigger. You might plan instead on taking a shower as soon as you get home and then starting dinner right away. The idea, obviously, is not to leave things to chance—plan exactly where you will be going within the house and what you will do there. Mindfully locate yourself in time and place—see the place, then follow through on your plan.

Keep your reasons for quitting close

Make a list—or even write a paragraph—of the most important reasons you have for overcoming your addiction. Write it in your Journal and keep it on hand. You can also attach a picture to it, say, of a loved one or a child or of a fitter, healthier you. When an overwhelming urge hits, it will try to push out thoughts of anything else. Having a reminder of your priorities where you can readily access it is a powerful way to put addictive cravings into perspective.

S.P.O.T. exercise

You will find this in Chapter 4, "Pause," on page 95, which describes being in the here and now so that you can identify and overcome addictive urges and cravings.

Meditate on your discomfort

Mindfulness meditation is a powerful, long-term anti-addiction practice, one that you have been working on throughout *Recover!*. It's also a terrific tool for combating urges as they arise, as I previewed in Chapter 3 on getting ready. There I discussed focusing your daily meditations on your breath or other ordinary parts of your existence. But you can also focus on more urgent feelings, like pain or discomfort. Craving is such a difficult feeling, one that can make you restless, agitated, even angry. One thing mindfulness teaches us is that feelings are not reality; they're not permanent. They're like clouds passing quickly across the sky.

Mindfulness Meditation: Suppressing Cravings

When you are in a suitable place to meditate and are relaxed, focus your attention on your craving and the feelings it creates for you: agitation, discomfort, longing, even emotional pain. As you focus your attention on these feelings, name them to yourself. You might say, "This is restlessness" or "This is frustration." And try to describe the quality of those feelings, how they present themselves in you—say you feel empty inside or, instead, a burning in your stomach. Notice, for instance, if you are fidgeting. You don't want to make these feelings go away, or to stop fidgeting. Just acknowledge that these things are present and real. Say to yourself, "This is how craving (or discomfort, or longing, etc.) feels right now." Concentrate on the feeling; notice how it shifts and mutates, how it is not always the same from one minute to the next. View this with a sense of curiosity, or with wonder.

Variation 1: Imagine your craving as a physical presence—ground undulating beneath you, or a wave that you are riding or surfing. Note that it varies in intensity. Ride up and down with the craving—note its high points and then how it declines.

Variation 2: Explore your body, and see if you notice any area that feels good or right—even if it is your nose or your feet. Focus your attention on that area, in the same way you would focus on your breath.

Variation 3: If you are feeling claustrophobic in your own skin—if you feel too agitated to relax at all—imagine expanding the space your body occupies, say, five inches all around you, and place your attention in that "free" space. Meditate in and from this place.

Variation 4: What is the happiest place you can imagine? Think about being there. Think of every sensory detail—see, hear, smell, taste, and touch these.

Variation 5: Imagine a ray gun. Visualize your craving as a robot or a monster. Then atomize it with your weapon. Imagine the robot or monster disintegrating, its pieces spraying all over the surrounding space, until it no longer has any substance. Or imagine the craving as an alien space ship that you're shooting at in a computer game with the same result.

Change your routine

Shake things up a bit! As it is, your life's routines are often structured around your addiction. Addiction *is* routine. You smoke, or eat, or drink, or use, or shop, or play games in the same places and times. So, do different things every day—or add things to your routine—that don't accommodate your addiction. Take a different route home from work, spend more time outside, talk to new people. Add a new thing every day or week.

What's the logical conclusion?

As I mentioned, addictive urges can overwhelm your ability to think clearly in the moment. When that little voice whispers to you that you could really use a [fill in the blank], it's difficult to see beyond the immediate gratification. Grab your PERFECT Journal and, in a section earmarked "cravings," work through the scenario: write down how it would feel to indulge your craving at this moment, but then follow this scenario through to its logical conclusion. If you start now, where will you be in a few hours? Will you feel bad and guilty almost immediately? Will you feel out of sorts, and tired, and sick in the morning? What are all the potential consequences? Be as detailed, as graphic, as possible.

Variation: If you find yourself actually experiencing the logical conclusion—say, you have just awakened with a mighty hangover—take the opportunity to write down everything you are feeling at the moment. Keep this record somewhere where you can easily refer to it.

Give yourself permission—for later

This technique might seem counterintuitive. But, white-knuckling your abstaining from your addiction, telling yourself that you will never, ever do it again, can be demoralizing in that it tends to increase your feelings of deprivation and hopelessness. In the last chapter I reviewed Roy Baumeister's research on willpower.[2] Your efforts at willpower can be exhausting and can get exhausted—it simply doesn't pay to bite off too much at once—or to intimidate yourself with what seem like insurmountable tasks ahead of you. Telling yourself that you're not going to do it now, but maybe another time, can release pressure. It's like a mental hack. It actually makes it less likely that you will indulge later. It works by giving you the feeling that you are in control, that you are making the decisions, thereby reinforcing your free will. The choice not to use is yours, and when you feel that it is a matter of choice, your priorities have a stronger voice, now and in the future.

Of course, AA tells people to focus "one day at a time." The essential difference with the mindfulness PERFECT Program approach is that AA actually means "forever." In PERFECT, you simply don't determine, don't limit who you are and will be forever. As we noted in Chapter 3, late in his life, the great Irish actor Richard Harris—after a major-league addictive history and a just-as-frequently recounted recovery—started having a Guinness stout or two at his local pub. As a grandfather in his seventies, Harris wasn't as driven to excess as he had been. AA and the disease theory, in having us view ourselves as permanently addicted, take advantage of a strange wrinkle in human thinking. We all recognize how much we have changed from the past to our present situation. Yet, when we project into the future, we imagine ourselves being very much the same as we are now. In fact, we are just as likely to change throughout our lives (that is, very likely), although we fail to recognize this future likelihood.[3]

Don't beat yourself up if you give in

In my discussions of conventional addiction treatment, harm reduction, and self-acceptance, I have emphasized that perfection is impossible and simple abstinence is not the gold standard. Believing that you are a lost cause simply because you fell off the wagon or are having a hard time getting on the wagon is unrealistic and self-destructive. If you have gone off the rails, treat yourself compassionately, learn from your experience as best you can, clean up the messes you've made, and—look forward. Your path is your own. No matter where you happen to be at the moment, you always have the choice and the chance to move forward.

Arrange social situations mindfully

Some people are more likely to be triggered by being alone, impelled by feelings of loneliness and boredom and resulting depression. For them, finding social outlets involving non-addicted others is crucial. But other addicts are set off when they are around other people. Quitting your addiction can feel more daunting when you are out with friends, or around people who are using when you are not—or trying not to.

First, let's get one boogeyman out of the way: Many people who are quitting an addiction worry about being conspicuous—calling undue attention to themselves—if they don't indulge. The truth is that most people don't notice and won't give it a second thought if you're not doing something. If you pass on a joint that's going around the room, they'll go on to the next person. If you don't have a cocktail in your hand, they won't ask you why. You don't owe anyone an explanation, and most people won't ask for one. Saying "no thanks" will usually garner a shrug. If you encounter some inappropriate outlier who lacks the good grace to ignore your abstinence, you can tell them that you're driving, training for a marathon, or pregnant (men—don't try this last one), and find someone else to talk to. There's no one you have to answer to about your choices.

Now, let's talk about more difficult situations—say you are with close friends who use your addictive object in a situation that you would normally spend indulging your addiction with them. If you are accustomed to or have often enjoyed doing something when you are with others, temptation can almost be irresistible when everyone else is partaking. Seeing other people do something that you might feel like doing can also make doing it seem less destructive. If they can do it, why can't you?

This is when your mindfulness skills and your clarity about your sense of purpose are key. Ask yourself whether and how your social circle supports your life values. It may be that your friends' only real connection to one another and to you is based on addiction. If you have nothing in common with a set of people aside from addiction, you might consider bowing out of that group and finding new friends. If people who have shared your addiction remain valuable to you, you can work on developing a deeper connection to some of them in situations that involve doing other things. Something as straightforward as deciding whom you will hang out with actually comprises an evidence-based therapy—one more often used in Great Britain than the United States—called "social behaviour and network therapy."[4]

It is not simply that friends and acquaintances of yours tend to be users themselves who tempt you to use—they may actually try to undermine your resolve to quit. Perhaps they miss their playmate or feel that your new direction is an indictment of their choices. It might even occur that someone close to you, who has been begging you to deal with your addiction, resents your quitting. So much of their life has been intertwined with your addiction—even simply through asking you to stop—that they find your abstinence intolerable! Or, it may be that they just don't trust you. You may also find people who don't believe that you can change your life if you are not in AA or NA and will not accept any other approach. Whatever the reason, you may find it difficult to gain support among your friends and family.

More basic relationships—such as within your family—can be the most challenging. Working through family relationships into sobriety will require your self-acceptance and compassion because those closest to you find it so difficult to trust and accommodate your change. They may respond to your new way of life with inexplicable anger—or even by discouraging or sabotaging you—often without recognizing what they are doing. For example, they may express pessimism that you can succeed, or they may even present triggers that they know set you off.

CASE: William's wife, Sabrina, was a stay-at-home mother who started drinking in the early afternoon. She was able to care for the household and the children, but was usually in bed by 9 p.m.—passed out. William was disgusted by her drinking and found the "wino housewife" routine so cliché. It was just not how he had envisioned his life with her when he proposed marriage. Sabrina had made many promises to William to stop, and tried several times. But, every time she tried, she would make it only a few days before William would start looking at her cynically, asking whether she had begun sneaking drinks again, or suggesting that she soon would be. With this lack of encouragement—actually, suspicion and cynicism—Sabrina's shaky willpower didn't last long.

So why would William undercut the very change he insists Sabrina needs to make by quitting drinking? While William is unhappy with his wife's lifestyle and its impact for him, he's also so used to it that he almost doesn't know who he is when he isn't martyring himself to Sabrina's addiction. Furthermore, he has built up reserves of resentment and distrust that are always ready to burst out of him. Putting down and doubting any gains Sabrina might claim she has made make him feel virtuous for all of his past suffering, and in an odd way give him control over the situation—which Sabrina's drinking likewise does. As long as she is drinking, he knows what to expect. When she stops, he does not, and that makes William deeply uncomfortable.

Let's say, however, that Sabrina has decided to end her destructive drinking, is clear about her reasons for doing so, and has shored up her inner resources and priorities. Of course, this is Sabrina's mission—she is the free-will protagonist in the terms of this book. But being married to and living with someone is a very challenging matter, on the one hand, and one that offers a great deal of potential support, on the other. William should be able to reinforce Sabrina's resolve, reward her efforts, and encourage her to go forward. He can be made aware (perhaps by reading this!) that he is undermining her instead. If he can clarify his purpose and goals—keeping them in line with Sabrina's, as they should be—he can be a very helpful resource for her quitting. And in doing so, he will be extending a welcome sense of compassion—including forgiveness for her past behavior that has hurt him—to the woman he loves. Because they should recognize that their marriage is the top priority for *both* of them, they should coordinate their efforts to make them both happier in a household without recrimination, belittling, and guilt. When each partner accepts that the other's efforts are genuine, together they can form a powerful team that will strengthen the two of them. William can then stop waiting for the other shoe to drop, or even trying to instigate Sabrina's failure.

Reciprocity marital counseling

Throughout this book I have emphasized the connection between the needs of an addict and his or her loved ones. Here is a place where the spouses' efforts need to be coordinated. The skills required for overcoming addiction are reciprocal ones.[5] One important alcoholism therapy that has repeatedly been shown to be among the most effective is called the community reinforcement approach, or CRA, which integrates changes throughout a person's work, recreational, and home life to reinforce sobriety.[6] One component of CRA is reciprocity marital counseling, in which two partners are led through a series of exercises where they share the importance of different aspects of their lives together (e.g., sexual, financial, child rearing) and how well these are being fulfilled. A counselor then assists the partners to see how their interlocking needs can be best satisfied by working cooperatively and by noting and rewarding positive changes each partner makes in the other's direction.

One of these areas, of course, is the addictive behavior. While couples sometimes find it awkward to engage in this counseling, they soon realize how positive the shifts can be for each of them and begin to "catch" and to appreciate their spouses doing good things for them—which itself puts their relationship on a new, positive footing.

Find professional help

Of course, CRA and reciprocity marital counseling are therapies that you'd have a hard time carrying out on your own. You can ask a competent marital counselor or therapist if they practice that type of treatment and undergo several sessions, always being clear when scheduling your next session that you expect it to add value, and ceasing when that isn't true. Likewise, addiction counseling by a sensible therapist or counselor can be a valuable aid. In keeping with the ideas underlying The PERFECT Program, you would seek out either a cognitive-behavioral therapist or a Buddhist psychologist, someone who is knowledgeable in mindfulness techniques. If you can't afford therapy, you can find free non-12-step groups such as SMART Recovery. (For links, see Chapter 10.) But you may also enlist a friend or family member you can rely on to help you with accountability.

Ask your friends for help

As you work toward achieving your life's vision, you may come up short when approaching certain arenas. Say you require babysitting so that you can attend a class, or maybe you need help organizing, learning to drive, using your computer, or cooking healthy meals. Ask your trusted friends and family for help. If, by chance, anyone declines your request, try not to take it personally or to consider it a rejection. They may have time constraints or other pressing obligations. But it is far more likely that they will be thrilled to share their knowledge or time with you, because they care about you, want to connect with you, and are proud to know they have something of value to offer toward your success.

Trusting that the people closest to you among your friends and family are willing to help you is difficult. It's hard to admit vulnerability to people you respect and to let people you care about really see the extent of your problems. It's possible you have been rebuffing them, or maybe you have imposed on or hurt them through your addiction. Furthermore, asking for help implies accountability to the people who are extending themselves for you. You might be afraid to disappoint them. But it is a sign of seriousness when you open yourself to this accountability by calling on your friends and family to ask for their help. And asking for and accepting their help allows them to show their love for you.

One word of caution: you may encounter people who will present you with ultimatums, or make intrusive or meddlesome demands of you in return for their help. This is a difficult scenario, especially when you are short on resources and feeling vulnerable. If you're presented with such a situation, you can shift your perspective to their point of view: Have you burned them in the past, and are they simply taking precautions? For example, if you request child care so that you can attend a class, and someone asks to see your registration or receipt first, rather than taking offense, see this as an opportunity to regain their trust. On the other hand, they may insist that you register for a program that they recommend, but that doesn't suit you, in return for their help. Hear them out, but make clear that in seeking their assistance you aren't turning your will and decision making over to them, or to anyone else.

Decision Making

Freedom from addiction is all about making choices, including individual daily decisions, dealing with problems, and global life planning. Effective decision making, problem solving, and goal setting require mindfulness, self-acceptance, and an awareness of your values, priorities, and purpose. As I discussed in the last chapter, it's easy to embark on—or fantasize about—an exciting new venture, but maintaining your drive is hard if you don't have a realistic vision of your strengths and what's actually possible for you, or the resources to support you when the going gets tough. Similarly, it's easy to make a self-destructive decision, in the moment, if your foundation is weak. If you have been following The PERFECT Program to this point, you should be in a better position than ever before to trust the choices you make for your future—you also have the skills you need to reassess your decisions and to rechart your course as needed. Finally, problem-solving techniques are learnable skills.

Perhaps you—like many people—are overwhelmed when you're confronted with situations requiring decisions. You may not trust yourself to make a good decision or don't believe that you are in a position to make decisions; perhaps you don't feel qualified or feel so stuck in your current circumstances that you don't have the freedom to *make* decisions. Such indecisiveness sometimes occurs because you believe your decision carries much more significance than it actually does and that tragic results can befall you no matter *which* way you decide. You may worry that your choices will expose something you want to hide. Consider the innocuous everyday example of a group of friends trying to decide where to go for lunch: No one wants to choose a place that will be disappointing, and so you'll hear a lot of, "Anywhere's fine! You decide." Or take a much more important decision, like "Should I ask for a divorce?" Making a decision is, essentially, taking a stand, asserting yourself and your will in line with your purpose, which can be nerve-wracking.

Having an addiction can make it much more difficult to make decisions, both because you have avoided making choices previously and because your addiction takes a lot of options off the table. As I have said, you adopt your addiction in good part as protection against the angst of decision making—you can *know* where you are headed without the effort or the pain of having to choose. Of course, the best way to develop the skill of choosing—like all skills—is practice. And every moment presents you with opportunities for choices. If you bring your mindful awareness to each opportunity, you will hone your ability to recognize when you have decisions to make and to choose directions that support your values, even in situations that trigger addictive urges.

CASE: Ralph was a partner in a seasonal business—it peaked when the school terms began, in September, January, and sometimes for summer school. During these periods, Ralph was under such intense pressure he could barely breathe. And what breaths he took were generally chemically infused. He took tranquilizers to stay calm, drank heavily after work, broke out into cigarette smoking, and got high on recreational drugs on the weekends. Yet, when each such period was over, he relaxed, sometimes at a beach home he enjoyed with his wife and kids. During these retreats, Ralph cut out virtually all his substance use (except for drinking wine after the kids were in bed). Yet he never used such reprieves to figure out new hires or how to rearrange responsibilities with his partners to fend off the wall of stress he inevitably faced around the corner, when he would once again succumb to all the pressures that caused his substance abuse.

By not addressing his work issues when he had a chance to, and by avoiding critical work-related decisions, Ralph was committing himself to perpetuating the unhealthy—dangerous—stress in his life and his resulting addictive behavior. And Ralph was a highly seasoned, successful professional.

JOURNAL: Write down decisions you have made in the last couple of days: decisions about people, at school or at work, etc. How many can you come up with? Did any of these decisions make you anxious? What insight do you have into why those decisions are more difficult than others? Then extend the scope of your deliberate, mindful decision making by identifying larger decisions over which you are hesitating, but that are important for you to make or that you will benefit from by making.

Problem solving

Problems are special events—often urgent—requiring your best decision making and coping. Your addiction is an example of faulty problem solving—of attempting to remove the pain or the awareness of a problem by using artificial means to mask it or to divert your attention. This process can involve either large problems (of the kind Rose faced in Chapter 1, where basic aspects of her life weren't working), persistent problems in one area (like Ralph's business tensions or a person's problems within a relationship or finding intimacy at all), or specific traumas or emergencies (such as failure of a relationship, or a financial or housing crisis, or an illness, or with a family member, like a child, and on down to smaller crises that can occur, sometimes several at once).

You may view life as a never-ending cascade of problems you must face off and deal with. This viewpoint can be excruciating, since it makes life so negative as to undermine the simple pleasures it offers, like taking time-outs, finding positive outlets, and enjoying people, activities, and the world. And such negativity often underlies the need to seek addictive escapes. On the other hand, the ability to cope with problems is an essential life skill, one that addicts as a group unfortunately often lack. Cognitive-behavioral psychologists teach people how to deal with problems directly, rather than turning to their addictions. The indexes of my earlier works, *Truth* and *Tools*, both point to sections that focus on this skill. The process involves five stages:

- **Recognize** you have a problem, that something is uncomfortable or hurting you.
- **Don't panic** but size up the matter, or slice it into manageable bits.
- **Seek information and inputs** from various sources, including solutions others have used.
- **Try out** one or several likely-seeming approaches.
- **Pause** after you have given an approach a fair shot, judge how well this effort has gone, and decide whether to continue in this mode or to try another approach.

The key to this process is to realize that problems occur, that you are not a special victim, and that you have the essential grasp, strength, and confidence to meet the challenge and emerge whole at the end. Life will go on, as will you.

Goal Setting

Your goals reflect what is important to you. Having goals keeps you on track, allows you to measure your progress, and infuses you with self-confidence and motivation, while driving you closer to your ultimate vision for yourself. Establishing realistic goals—meaning that they are achievable, that they are what you genuinely want, and that they jibe with your strengths and values—is an art that requires you to set priorities based on your values and a true understanding of yourself and your capacities. In Chapter 3, you completed the Goals Worksheet. For your convenience, I present the worksheet again. Please review your earlier answers and update them as you see fit. You'll notice that the worksheet follows a certain outline, beginning with a grand vision for yourself and ending with a manageable to-do list of things you can accomplish right away to get the ball rolling.

GOALS WORKSHEET

1. Long-Term Goals

a. Visualize your ideal life and write about it in as much detail as possible. You might describe what a typical day of freedom looks like, for example.

2. Short-Term Goals

a. On one line, name three areas of your life that are suffering because of your addiction and, under each one, list some possible changes you can make right now to spark improvement in those areas.

b. Read over your options—some of them will be ambitious and some will be practical. Choose the one change from each list that seems most doable to you. For instance, if you are sedentary and concerned about your health, choosing to train for a 5K might sound inspiring, but a more realistic goal might be to start walking three times a week.

c. Now, under each of your choices, make note of things that will help you achieve these goals. To continue with the example above, what would you need to begin walking? A pair of sturdy but comfortable shoes? Some motivating music queued up on your MP3 player? A walking schedule? A walking buddy? A dog (you can always borrow a neighbor's, and your neighbor will thank you)? Begin gathering your resources.

d. Set a day to start implementing each of these changes, and set up a tracking system. You can use a calendar, a daily checklist, or your PERFECT Journal. There are even websites out there (like http://www.43things.com) that help you set goals, track your progress, and connect with others who share your goals. A free online calendar, like Google or Yahoo, will allow you to send reminders to yourself.

e. Remember that making these changes points you in the direction of true recovery. You are aligning yourself with your values. If you miss a day or slack off, just pick the ball back up. Every moment is an opportunity to make a positive choice.

3. Mid-Range Goals

a. Consider the journal entry you wrote on your vision for yourself, and make a list of goals you will need to meet to actualize your vision. For example, if you see yourself earning a degree, you will need to begin researching programs and requirements. Do you have to earn your GED or take the GRE?

b Are there things you can do right now to begin preparing? If not, when would be a realistic time to begin? Write down that date.

4. Addiction Goals

Taking all your answers into consideration, and recalling from Chapter 3—perhaps rereading the various options presented there—what is your ultimate goal in regard to the substance or behavior you are addicted to? What is the best way for you to achieve that? For instance, if you are aiming for abstinence, is it more realistic *for you* to taper off, to implement harm reduction methods, or to go cold turkey? If you are aiming for moderation, is that a long-term goal that you expect you will fall short of sometimes in the present? If so, how will you handle your addiction while protecting yourself in the meantime? Compose a plan for yourself now, listing your addiction goals and the avenue you want to take there. Be as cooly realistic as you can be. Remember, you can always go back and revise your plan as you gain clarity about yourself and your values.

Coping Skills

Now, let's drill down even farther into the specific areas of your life that may have been neglected or dissolved into overwhelming disarray as you were absorbed in addiction. As we mature, we tend to learn life skills organically, through observation and practice, trial and error. We develop habits and systems—and, depending on our personalities, we may be adept in some areas while we struggle through others. Someone may be a wizard of efficiency at work, but completely disorganized at home.

That's normal. When you're emerging from addiction, however, you might find yourself completely stymied by all of it, not having developed global skills or resources (remember how many aspects of her life Rose, in Chapter 1, had to tackle at one time?). Let's bring your self-acceptance, the self-awareness you have gathered, and the basics of goal setting and decision making to the following arenas and get started putting things in order.

Remember that you will be more inspired and adept in some areas, while others will seem more tedious and unimportant. That's okay. It's the rare person who can maintain a perfect sense of balance. Even Martha Stewart couldn't keep her financial life in order. So, be gentle with yourself. Since an entire book could be written on each of these subjects (and they have been), I will offer you an overview and, in Chapters 8 and 10, will provide further ideas and resources. This is a starting place. Begin by completing your Goals Worksheet, 1 through 3, for each area. You may find that your goals have become clearer or better developed since you filled out the worksheet in Chapter 3.

Communication Skills: Listening

Paying attention to others is difficult when your mind is focused elsewhere—like on your addiction or what's next on your to-do list. Or, let's be honest, when the subject doesn't interest you because it isn't about you. Genuinely listening when someone is talking to you takes effort and a certain generosity of spirit that improves with practice. It may seem obvious that listening is a good thing to do, but be clear about why that is: First of all, when someone feels that you are honestly paying attention to what they're saying, it makes them feel important. Sometimes, listening to someone is more about establishing and reinforcing the foundation of your relationship than about what they are saying at that moment. It doesn't matter if you're riveted by the subject matter. Second, it inspires a feeling of trust and goodwill toward you—people will continue to seek out your company. Third, listening is a good way to practice your mindfulness skills. Bringing your attention to someone else—even when you're not fascinated—is the essence of mindfulness. Fourth, you might learn something about your conversation partner or about yourself if you are listening rather than simply waiting for them to stop talking so that you can start. You may feel that you are not being interesting enough if you aren't constantly talking, but the truth is that people will feel that *you* are interesting when you make *them* feel interesting.

Listening is the single most important skill for therapists to cultivate. Some common ways of developing *your* listening skills (some of which you may already be familiar with) are these: Sometimes simply repeating what the other person has said will reassure them that you are attentive and concerned. "Mirroring" means rephrasing or interpreting what you have just heard and offering it back to your companion so they can elaborate. For example, if someone is sharing something personal with you, you can say, "It must have been shocking to learn that your mother has been keeping such a dark secret." Here you are reflecting the emotions the situation created for your friend.

You might also expand and interpret something he or she has said. "It seems to me that what your mother did has really been upsetting to you even today, all these years later!" You can see the big difference between such reflective comments and saying, "My cousin's mother had a secret, too." Other listening techniques include thinking of questions you can ask to move the conversation along. Ask for more detail; ask about how the person felt about an event; ask them what insights they gathered from it. These are essential methods used in the cognitive-behavioral technique called *motivational interviewing* or *motivational enhancement*, which I discuss below, in which the therapist constantly turns the interaction back to the individual seeking help to allow them to develop their insights and to spark and focus their motivation to change something that is causing them difficulty.

Emotional Skills

Patience and choosing your battles

Of course, listening requires patience. But sometimes you may find that certain people or social situations aggravate you. For instance, suppose you are in a hurry at the grocery store and end up in line behind a customer who doesn't speak English, doesn't understand the payment system, or can't find her money. It's taking forever. You might want to throw a body-language tantrum by tapping your foot, sighing, looking at your watch. You might even want to grab her wallet out of her hand and get her money out for her. You then fume about it all the way home. Life throws us curve balls all the time, usually in the form of other people. We have to wait for them, wait on them, accommodate them, drive behind them, work for them, answer their phone calls, and deal with their idiosyncrasies and ignorance. That's what it means to get along in this world. And, in no small way, life is an accumulation of such moments, as is your overall mood. Allowing for this human truth will make your life much more peaceful. Consider that, in pursuing your addiction, you may have tried people's patience yourself!

Maintaining your perspective is the key to patience, starting with the Buddhist or universalist insight that we are all part of a large, moving universe, human and otherwise. Try to keep in mind that a lot is going on at all times outside of your small realm. Not everyone is on your schedule; not everyone knows the things you know; people make mistakes in traffic (including you). Say you're back in that grocery line, waiting for your turn behind the frustrating customer who is taking a lifetime at the counter. Be aware that, no matter how long it takes her to figure it out, you will surely have your turn within mere minutes. Imagine, as well, her own frustration or embarrassment, especially if she is not fluent in the language—going shopping takes some guts! Take into account that, if you are in a rush, you might have managed your time better. And finally, what is the absolute worst that will happen if she takes another five minutes to count out her bills? Losing your patience is something you can control (a topic for the next chapter).

JOURNAL: Write down some of the scenarios that you know cause you to lose your patience: Having to explain something more than once? Seeing the toilet paper turned the wrong way on the roll? Friends who are always late? Drivers who don't use their turn signal? When you examine this list, can you decide which items are irrelevant and which ones you might find ways to mitigate? Are there some over which you have no control, but others that you can't—or shouldn't—tolerate? Are there situations you contribute to or condone by not speaking up? We often lose our patience about things we could exert some control over. Take, for example, the perpetually late friend. He is always twenty minutes late. This is a battle worth picking, because your schedule is as important as his. Think about realistically changing *that*. Seething silently or lashing out with passive-aggressive barbs instead is not effective, and the scenario will simply repeat itself.

Mindfulness: Curing Road Rage

Consider what you are doing when you get angry at some stranger for some misdeed—or imagined misdeed—on the highway or the street before you. You are deciding that this person—idiot, miscreant, or innocent that he or she is—can affect your nervous system and brain and significantly alter your view of the universe and mood for the day. My, that's a big consequence to your life from someone's not signaling a turn! How does that unsignaled turn stack up against your precarious financial position, wayward child, or conflicted marriage or intimate relationship, let alone global warming, the national debt, and our troops fighting and dying around the world? I'm sorry to bring all of those up! But you get the point—what this bad driver did is **nothing**.

If there's one thing you can count on, it's that every day you will be presented with opportunities to navigate obstacles: Your kids will break something; there will be road construction at rush hour; there will be yet another form to fill out; customer service will give you the runaround. Not allowing these things to bug you isn't always easy, and sometimes you just have to stomp around about it. But you don't want to be the type of person who comes unglued at the slightest hitch in things. *Because these are peak moments for resorting to—or else, relapsing back into—an addiction.*

There are some things you can't anticipate, but can use your loving kindness skills and mindfulness to achieve perspective about. Some things you can anticipate: put your Ming vase in the cupboard until the kids are grown; leave home earlier and bring a good audiobook for the ride; read the directions carefully and ask questions; ask to speak with a more helpful representative. Finally, bring your self-knowledge and priorities to bear in cases that require you to negotiate with other people.

Know—and be true to—yourself

It might seem that having social skills means being popular, having a lot of friends, holding court, being witty and attractive. And that a quiet person who avoids crowds, prefers the company of close friends, or would rather engage in solitary activities is lacking in social skills. Neither is true. Social skills are simply your ability to navigate as a worthy person among people in your life in a way that is true to you, so that you and others can coexist peacefully and develop productive and satisfying relationships. And most of us fall somewhere in the range between introvert and extrovert. *When you consider your vision for your life, ask yourself if it matches what you know to be true about yourself.* Do you imagine yourself having a packed social calendar, when in fact you may really enjoy having a cup of coffee with a friend once in a while? Or, do you imagine yourself living a life of quiet contemplation, gardening or knitting or meditating on a mountaintop, when you really love to be around other people, at least periodically? Do you find yourself feeling drained after an outwardly enjoyable event with other people? Or do such situations energize you? Would you rather play a team sport or a sport in which you are competing only with yourself?

EXERCISE: Contemplate your idea of social life. Do you see yourself engaging with people in a way that you are currently not doing? For instance, if you are mostly solitary, do you envision a life surrounded by friends? If you are overly involved with people, do you see yourself spending more time alone? Keeping in mind that it is not better to be either an extrovert or an introvert (can you think of an objective reason why one is preferable?), which do you think describes you best? If you enjoy a lot of company, but would like to spend more time alone, can you think of activities you can engage in that will introduce more solitude into your life without abandoning your social life? For instance, you might consider taking up a new activity with one other person, or choosing something you can do on your own. If you spend most of your time alone, but would like to be more involved socially, can you think of activities that will bring you around people, but that will not be overwhelming? You might join a walking group, for instance, or take a class.

Being comfortable in your own skin is one of life's greatest challenges, and rewards—as Chapter 5, on self-acceptance, describes. As in other areas, your mindfulness skills will help you achieve a clear perspective to guide you in assessing and navigating your social life. Being able to recognize when you are expecting the impossible from yourself or beating yourself up for not meeting arbitrary standards is a skill you can develop.[7]

And, of course, being true to yourself does not mean hurting other people in order to satisfy your newly realized emotions. Just because you have decided it is time to assert yourself does not justify offloading against friends, relatives, or the smoothie clerk (as Steve Jobs often did).

Appreciating others' successes

When Warren was in the first grade, he started taking Kung Fu with a group of other kids his age. A few times a year some members of the class who excelled at a particular level would be elevated a rank, in the company of their classmates, who would then shake hands and bow to the kids who had received this honor. Warren was always thrilled when he was up for a new rank, but felt destroyed and despondent when other kids would elevate. He couldn't see that other kids' elevation was not a personal insult directed at him or a put-down of his abilities. Whenever he came sulking out of class after watching his classmates earn a new stripe on their belts, Warren's mother would ask him how he would feel if the other kids responded as grudgingly when it was his turn to elevate. "Do you want them to be happy for you or mad at you?" After continuing in his Kung Fu for a few more years, Warren's perspective gradually changed. Watching his peers progress according to their skills, while he continued to move up as well, allowed him to genuinely appreciate being part of the celebration—part of his community of classmates—no matter who was receiving the honor. It taught him to recognize that his pace is his own, but also allowed him to view his friends' successes as inspiration and motivation.

Feeling genuine joy for others' accomplishments in life is not natural to everyone—maybe not to most people. Do you know the term *schadenfreude*?[8] For many—or most—of us, taking delight in others' misfortunes makes us feel better about ourselves, since we judge ourselves by comparing our fates with others'. This is more true the less secure our own footing is.[9] It takes an effort of will and a deliberate shift in perspective to turn your focus away from yourself and toward someone else in a positive way. One of our national pastimes is to invade celebrities' lives, following them around with a microscope, picking their lives apart in minute detail: their wardrobe choices, their bodies, their relationships. Clearly, this satisfies some collective urge to bring others low, even if they have no relationship to us. It's also something we do to each other on a personal level, as when we direct resentment or spread gossip about people who seem to have something we don't, or feel jealousy rather than joy at a co-worker's wedding announcement or promotion.

Not only do these practices diminish your sense of well-being and integrity, they also shift your attention from your accomplishments and strengths. On the one hand, worrying about other people's successes and failures really has no consequences for—and may actually impede—getting into the swing of your own life. Furthermore, being able to celebrate and respect others for what they have or what they are doing—or, alternately, feeling compassion when they fail—connects you to people in a positive way. Anything that enhances your feeling of community, of belonging, is good for you. Just as they did for young Warren, others' accomplishments can inspire and motivate you.

Boundary Setting

Respecting boundaries—yours and others'

The notion of maintaining one's boundaries hit the mainstream a long time ago, but its meaning can be vague and self-serving. For some, it means taking an uncompromising stand or putting yourself first in all circumstances; for others, it means learning to say "no"—important, but still just one part of the picture. Respecting boundaries requires you to know your own limits, and also to know whether it's appropriate to be flexible or to stand firm. It also means recognizing and respecting others' boundaries, without taking their limits as personal affronts. You deserve to be treated respectfully, whatever your quirks, and it is your job—no one else's—to make sure others don't demean or discount you. The converse requires that you don't pressure others to act outside their comfort zone—even when you believe it may be best for them. Here are a few basic elements in respecting boundaries:

- **Defining your boundaries:** What lines won't you cross? For example, will you never drink or smoke or take drugs in front of your parents or your child? Equally important in setting boundaries is what you will refuse to allow others to do to you, or even in your presence. Actions, activities, or behaviors that make you uncomfortable or that you will not tolerate from other people because they compromise your values or detract from your quality of life form such boundaries. If you have friends who indulge in malicious gossip about other members of your circle, perhaps you think they are behaving badly. But you can get caught up in the moment and listen or participate, despite your unease. Setting your boundaries in cases like this can be difficult because you fear rejection from your friends, perhaps becoming the next topic of conversation. How might you draw a line so as not to violate your values in a situation like this?

- **Knowing how to be flexible without violating your values:** Can you make exceptions to your rules, if, for instance, it would serve a higher purpose? Can you do so without feeling undermined? Other types of boundaries include how you respond to requests (or demands) from others. Suppose you have a family member whom you love, but who has consistently taken advantage of you, and lately you have steadfastly denied her requests. She is currently in need of help. You have values in conflict: On one hand, you want to avoid feeling used; yet you feel her suffering. Can you think of ways you might help her without compromising your integrity, perhaps by imposing clear limits on, or conditions for, your help?
- **Effectively and respectfully communicating your boundaries:** Are you able to tell people directly when their behavior violates your boundaries? Can you do so before you are feeling helpless or angry? Are you afraid of what will happen if you draw a line in the sand? What if a friend ignores crosswalks and sends pedestrians scurrying while you, as a bicyclist, are hypersensitive about respecting people who aren't in cars and trucks? Are you sure to mention to your friend that you feel they are doing something wrong? How sternly should you make your point? Should you refuse to drive with them if they keep it up; to stop dealing with them altogether? What if a friend talks to counter servers—or to his or her children, for that matter—in a disrespectful way? Will you bring it up to your friend? If so, immediately or later? How will you introduce the topic?
- **Being clear about the consequences of violating your boundaries:** Clearly communicating your boundaries is part of the broader question: How will you respond if someone violates

your boundaries? Are you clear with yourself and others about those consequences? Will you follow through? Children are perhaps the most skillful boundary pushers on earth: Say you are at the store with your child, who is making your shopping trip impossible by begging and crying for toys and candy. And you respond by alternately pleading for cooperation, issuing threats, and giving in. Now, imagine telling your child, before you enter the store, that if they begin whining and pleading, you will pick them up, walk out of the store, and give them a time-out at home. And imagine actually doing so, matter-of-factly, without losing your cool. You know that if you are consistent with your response, your child will learn quickly. Are there other areas of your life where this approach will serve you well? One that we discuss below, with CRAFT, involves children or spouses who violate the sanctity of the family or household through their drug use or drinking.

- **Learning to reassess or redefine your boundaries based on experience:** What if you realize that a boundary you have been protecting is no longer relevant to you? Can you change or discard that boundary? Sometimes, for example, you feel that you must cut off contact with a person who has hurt you in the past, especially if you are vulnerable to being hurt by them again. A lot of healing and growth can happen over time (per Chapter 5, about children who come to or are considering forgiveness of parents who have neglected or abused them). You might find that, while there was a time when a certain person held some negative power over you, they no longer do. Whether or not they have changed or are remorseful, *you* are no longer vulnerable to being hurt by them, or you have forgiven them. It might be time to reconsider your boundary, especially if you genuinely care about them or have other reasons to reconnect.
- **Understanding that others deserve the same rights:** How do you respond when someone denies your request for help? In the first place, what are reasonable requests for you to make of your friends and family? When someone denies your request, your feelings will almost surely be hurt. However, can you also take

a perspective that allows you to accept such decisions as not being a comment on your value to those you know and love, but more one based on their personal circumstances? In other words, can you remove yourself as the presumed primary factor in others' personal choices?

Standing up for yourself

The best known, most often used method for respecting boundaries is assertiveness training, which teaches people to express their needs and preferences calmly, firmly, and respectfully. At one extreme is complete passivity and submissiveness, where a person makes no effort to be clear about his or her values or wishes. At the other extreme is open aggressiveness, where people impose their values and requirements on others with no regard for others' feelings, values, or needs. Assertiveness takes a constructive stance between these extremes.

Assertiveness includes being able to give and receive feedback. When you feel that your boundaries are being violated, both in terms of your basic values and in your addictive areas, you need tools to allow you to tell others where your boundaries are and how they may be overstepping them. In doing so, you need to rely on communication—or feedback—skills. Here are key elements of giving people feedback about your boundaries:

- Be specific about what you don't like and explain why you don't like it: that is, how it violates your boundaries or values.
- Don't express anger or dislike toward the person/people, but only at the behavior or the message of which you disapprove.
- Reinforce your liking or love of the person or people (if this is true) to whom you are giving the feedback.
- Describe what you need to take place in order to continue in the interaction/relationship.

One further element in the feedback process is that you need to be able to accept and respond in the same vein to feedback others give you when you violate their values or overstep their boundaries. Suffice it to say, you want to be as open to their sincere expression of their concerns as you hope they will be to yours.

Boundaries and Addiction Treatment

Helping others

Boundary maintenance is important when giving as well as receiving feedback. What if people don't respond to the wisdom you offer them? Can you respect that their expectations and desires may simply be different from yours? Or that they simply are not prepared to make changes, even when you may be right that these would be good for them? Of course, addiction often drives a person's relatives and friends around the bend, causing them to become more and more forceful in their demands, to the point of constraining the addict's options and behaviors. In the law, this is permissible when the person becomes a danger to themselves and/or others. But in any but extreme circumstances, taking control of someone else's life out of their hands has serious implications, some of which you may never be able to reverse.

Boundary violations in addiction treatment

The belief that addiction means that a person cannot control themselves, and that addictive behavior inevitably leads to decline, collapse, and ultimately death, has been used to justify all sorts of unwanted intrusions into people's lives. Taking this approach more often than not backfires and doesn't produce positive results.[10] The hectoring that goes on in 12-step circles is considered sacred because its practitioners claim, "We know what you are better than you do" (remember that Rose, in Chapter 1, had this experience). Violating someone else's personal space and autonomy includes taking away their right to their own self-conception. After all, when people say, "I don't believe I am a lifelong addict," they are far more often right than wrong—especially when they are young. Yet young people are those most likely to receive such unrestrained—even vicious—attacks on their own self-definitions and wills. Tough Love is one example of unrestrained boundaries in the addiction treatment industry that has been shown to do much more harm than good, both with adolescents and with adults.[11]

Accepting those close to you

When someone close to you is self-destructive, you naturally want to help. Presenting people you love with ultimatums or cutting them out of your life completely can go against your most life-affirming instincts. That is not to say that there are not times when you must do so. As we have seen, people are often acting in some sense of their own interest by pursuing addictive gratifications and, for some, this may be the best they are capable of at the time. Ultimately, most become clear about better ways to find satisfaction and get what they need from life. In the meantime, whether or not you decide to close the door on a relationship requires you to prioritize your values and to know yourself and what you can live with. It is an extreme scenario, one that requires you to maintain your boundaries—say, with a child or a spouse—in day-to-day life, as described above. This means:

- Accepting the people and situations into your life that bring you fulfillment and satisfaction, even if they are difficult or challenging.
- Excluding the people and situations that detract from or compromise your priorities, or that do you or your loved ones actual harm.
- When there is no simple answer, moderating or accommodating your demands, but withdrawing as required at particular moments, in a way that allows you to maintain your integrity.

Effective Therapies

Community reinforcement and family training (CRAFT)

Recover! tells you that you can get over an addiction on your own, as most people do. It offers you information in a non-technical form that you can use yourself and in the service of others. Yet, some people don't get better, or at least at the pace you need them to in order for you to be content in your own life and on their behalf. What do you do when a family member's or loved one's addiction is disturbing, disrupting, or hurting you and the rest of the family? The alternatives include trying to be as helpful as you can be or, if you're in a position to do so, to help or encourage the person to find an effective treatment.

I have interspersed in this chapter references to cognitive-behavioral therapy techniques. One such resource is called Community Reinforcement and Family Training, or CRAFT,[12] which is an extension of the Community Reinforcement Approach (CRA) described above. As with other such techniques, I review CRAFT in *Truth* and *Tools*. Here I describe its basic concepts. CRAFT is a way of applying behavioral reinforcement techniques within a family context. It aims to teach spouses and parents how to (1) protect themselves and other family members, particularly children, and (2) encourage addicted family members to seek needed help for themselves. CRAFT's elements are simply extensions of the boundary principles already discussed:

- Be clear on your own boundaries, needs, and self-protection. Make these limits crystal clear to an addicted family member, and allow them to participate in the family so long as they observe these boundaries.
- Be prepared to expel the family member—either temporarily or for a longer duration—when they refuse, or fail, to honor the boundaries.
- Access and make the family member aware of help they can seek (for example, therapy) in order to help themselves and potentially reenter the family context.

One form of addiction treatment you may be aware of from television is interventions, in which severely addicted people are confronted with an absolute need to seek treatment—which they are then forced into. Judging from the great successes TV portrays, you might wonder why every addict in the world isn't simply coerced to attend treatment as these fortunate souls were. Well, aside from the violations of personal integrity and potential legal violations I have discussed, these interventions simply don't work well (which is often apparent even in the shows that promote them). One of the best known of these, *Celebrity Rehab*, administered by Dr. Drew Pinsky, attracted a lot of negative attention when Mindy McCready became the fifth of the show's alumni to die.[13] Most people don't end up succeeding when they're forced into treatment (nearly always 12-step, of course).[14] In fact, most don't even end up going. CRAFT is an alternative that has been shown superior for helping the addicted family member, whether or not treatment is ultimately involved.[15]

CASE: Riva's boyfriend Glenn abused alcohol, and it often made him unreliable and ugly. They had a young child together. Riva's constant fear was that the boy would see—or just sense—Glenn's problem drinking, and that it would affect the boy both directly and indirectly. Yet she was reluctant to throw Glenn out of the home. For one thing, as the father of her child, she couldn't ever completely get rid of him.

Riva went to a therapist who she heard was good in such situations. Together, they made a list of behaviors that Riva simply would no longer tolerate—and she would lock Glenn out of the house when he did these—getting a restraining order if necessary to do so.

On the other hand, Riva wanted to offer Glenn every chance to reenter their home and participate fully so long as he wasn't drinking (or drinking in an ugly manner). She and the therapist she saw also drew up a list of likely resources—support groups, from AA to SMART Recovery, as well as potential counselors, men's groups, anger management classes, etc.—for Glenn to access, if he thought these would help him meet the mark that Riva was now setting for him.

Motivational interviewing

Perhaps the single most difficult skill discussed here is learning how to assist people without telling them what they should do. The first skill I trained all my counselors at my residential treatment center to use was a listening technique called "motivational interviewing" or "motivational enhancement," as developed by William Miller and his colleagues.[16] People don't respond when you instruct them on how to act—even when they ask you to tell them exactly that. Instead, addiction clients—like everybody—react defensively when given such instructions, which, of course, people take to be criticisms. People argue back, even counterattack, thinking: "They just don't understand me and my situation."

And people—you—are right. No one can understand your needs, goals, and situation as you can; nor can you understand any other person's as well as they can. Therefore, as Miller and other researchers have shown, the best way to encourage the motivation to change—and actual changes—is to help people come to grips with their problems through their own thinking and motivational processes. You enable others to do this—as I have discussed above—by listening and with sympathetic, genuinely inquisitive questioning, a process called motivational interviewing (MI). MI is currently the most popular therapy technique in addiction circles. Just about every program claims to use it, even when it is the last thing counselors and the program believe in. As Anne Fletcher demonstrated in her book *Inside Rehab* (Viking, 2013), addiction counselors and programs actually rarely use effective approaches like MI. Most such programs and counselors instead follow a top-down, dictatorial model. If they did use MI, they would have to permit the addict to pursue whichever path he or she feels is likely to work best, including moderation or harm reduction, as long as that is their preferred route (which they are therefore going to pursue anyhow).

The Questioning Exercise

The next time someone—a friend or family member—asks you for advice, tell them that before you can offer them any inputs, you first need to clarify their situation for yourself. Then question them. Some key elements you might cover are:

- Information about the person: their backgrounds, experiences, current situation (job, family, emotional).
- Only after establishing these personal foundations—including your willingness and ability to listen sympathetically—ask them to flesh out the problem that concerns them, whether addictive or otherwise.
- During the course of the above, ask the person what is most important to them (family, work, health, self-determination, religion, whatever) and how this affects the problem—and, specifically, why it makes them want to change (remember the case of Ozzie in Chapter 2, who decided to quit smoking when someone made him realize it directly opposed his union allegiance).
- Without ever presenting your own views directly, work as best you can through your questioning to explore the person's expressed reasons

for changing and the consequences they have experienced from their problem (addictive or otherwise), allowing them to make as many and as vivid connections as they can between what is important to them and the need for change.

This is the therapy that has most demonstrated its effectiveness in the case of addiction, and much else.

Moving Forward

This chapter has given you a lot to digest. Take a moment to pause, reflect, meditate. When you're ready, we will move on and devote the next chapter to putting your skills and values into action and to achieving balance in your life through self-awareness and reframing your perspective on failure.

CHAPTER 8

Embark

Equilibrium—Proceeding on an even keel

CHAPTER GOALS

- To develop a foundation of self-knowledge
- To decide what to change and what to do now
- To take first steps into your new life
- To understand and prevent relapse

Purpose: Preparing for a journey, while necessary, is a lot of work: charting your course, honing your skills, gathering your resources, anticipating challenges and troubled waters. It's possible to spend a lifetime planning and arranging and waiting for the perfect moment to shove off. Ultimately, there is no perfect time, and no amount of preparation can be as valuable to you as the lessons you learn and the skills you develop by actually doing. This chapter is devoted to encouraging you to set sail and guiding you through some of the early demands on you and rough patches that may shake your resolve. Above all, you want to keep your forward motion, which requires—and also helps you maintain—your balance. This requires sharpening your self-knowledge or awareness, so that you can make deliberate choices based on your priorities; acting decisively on the decisions you make; and being able to maintain your larger perspective through failure and relapse by treating them as information to learn from.

Self-Knowledge and Personal Choice

Learning about yourself—developing insights into who you are, what you want, how you function—is self-knowledge (or self-awareness). Self-knowledge is a critical skill in fighting addiction. There is no one approach to overcoming addiction, and The PERFECT Program is designed to help you discover a path that honors your heart, values, and personal choices. Your goal is not simply to quit your addiction, but to make addiction impossible by replacing it with a path of your own design that is true to you. Knowing yourself, your strengths and passions as well as your vulnerabilities and areas of self-deception, is essential both for making on-the-spot decisions and for completing your long-term goals. Self-knowledge is the engine of free will; it allows you to understand your motivations and then to make decisions consciously and deliberately, with your purpose in mind. Addiction generates a massive blind spot, preventing you from seeing beyond its own immediate satisfaction. Whether or not you have been addicted to anything, you surely have witnessed the results of this blind spot in other people. Perhaps you have even expressed frustration and incredulity over their unwillingness to see what is so clear to everyone else: "Why doesn't she leave him?" "What was he thinking when he did that?" "How could she leave her kids alone?" "Who does such a thing?" And, maybe you offer a concession to your own blind spot, "I have my moments, but I'd *never* go that far." You probably *wouldn't* go that far, and you know yourself well enough to make that assertion.

CASE: Liam is strikingly handsome—compelling in a rakish, movie-star kind of way. He is also a long-term alcoholic. His friends (of whom there are few) and acquaintances commonly refer to him as "a drunk"—if not worse. "Drunk" is a harsh term, but the images it conjures are apt for this person. Liam is, it seems to everyone, a lost cause. Insufferable and obnoxious, he blows the fuse on everyone's last nerve and has been banned from almost every bar in town. He wears out his welcome almost instantly by telling racist and sexist jokes, making rude observations about other patrons, and—like the classic drunk—spilling his drinks and falling off his stool.

Although Liam seemingly has no limits and no restraint, there are two things he will not do no matter how impaired he is: He will not drive drunk, and he will not cheat on his girlfriend (surprisingly, Liam does indeed have a longtime girlfriend).

Liam's personal taboos—few in number as they may be—are deeply ingrained in him. They spring from genuine values: his sense of loyalty to his companion and his unwillingness to chance hurting or killing someone. No matter how wasted he may be and no matter how many bridges he burns or people he offends, he is incapable of giving himself permission to cross those certain lines. The converse of Liam's case is also true. Excusing poor behavior by blaming it on addiction is one of the ways that addiction blinds—or deludes—us. After reading Liam's story, you might say, for instance, "Okay, so maybe I drive occasionally when I'm high, but I'd never tell a racist or sexist joke no matter how messed up I get." If you had a similar thought, ask yourself this question: "How is it that, no matter how impaired I am, I will never do one thing, but can still find an excuse to do the other?" It's really rather remarkable, when you think about it.

Consider, for example, someone who is prone to flying into rages. He's unpredictable, and people walk on eggshells around him, never sure what will set him off or when he will throw a tantrum. When this guy loses it, he screams obscenities, slams doors, stomps around, menacing and invading others' personal space. He might throw something across the room or turn over a piece of furniture or put his fist into the wall. When it's all over with, he always feels ashamed of himself and excuses his behavior by saying that he was so angry that he lost control. If you were brave, you could ask him at this point, "If you're so out of control, how come you haven't killed anyone yet?" Think about it like this: even when this loose cannon is in a blind rage, he is always able to prevent himself from taking his behavior to the point of no return. From where does that self-control and will come?

This example and Liam's case are both extreme and disturbing scenarios. I have included them here to demonstrate that everyone—no matter how far gone—has standards and lines they will not cross. The taboos they have established for themselves spring directly from their personal priorities. But the converse is also true. Say you do things that you feel violate your true value system as a result of your addiction, such as cheat on your partner while drunk, gamble away your children's college fund, or skip work to play World of Warcraft. It's a difficult pill to swallow—but you would not do these things if you did not give yourself permission to.

Self-knowledge is a lifelong process of discovery. Shedding light on your motivations requires you to bring your self-acceptance practice to bear on everything you learn about yourself. You might find that you have certain positive priorities that you always honor. Say, for instance, you haven't yet quit smoking, but you never smoke in the house or in front of children. Or, although you have a serious drinking problem, you never drink too much while with your parents. Clearly, your commitment to your family is key and inviolable. But you may find that other values you hold dear are more easily shunted to the wayside—your own health, for instance.

To continue with the example of the smoker, let's say there are a couple of value systems in conflict within you. Smoking provides you with some alone time, helps you focus on your work, and makes you feel productive. At the same time, you know that you're putting your health at risk through your smoking and thereby endangering your family's well-being. How do you reconcile this? When you allow yourself to see that you have a conflict of values, you are in a position to make some decisions, to act on your primary motivations. Rage-aholics who are able to control their behavior despite being consumed by anger seem to do so in unplanned ways. That is, they don't deliberate about which acts of violence they will commit. They're acting on autopilot. Self-knowledge allows you to shine light on the motivations behind these choices, hidden somewhere within you, so that you can make your decisions intentional ones.

Here are exercises and practices that will help you become more self-aware:

BE PRESENT: As I discussed in Chapter 4, we all experience moments of grace, in which we hear from our inner self. Rather than waiting for these moments to arise spontaneously, call them forth deliberately. Whenever it occurs to you—perhaps set a chime on your cell phone as a reminder a few times a day or choose a regular time every day, say, when you're in the shower—to stop what you're doing for a couple of minutes and bring your attention into the present moment and to all your senses. What are you doing at the moment? How is your posture? What is the quality of light in the room or outside? What are the objects that surround you? What do you hear? Smell? Do you have any aches or pains? What is your mood? You don't have to write anything down. Just notice, and bring yourself as fully into the present as possible.

MOVE: If you are a physically active person, employ the same "Being present" exercise when you are engaged in an activity. Bring your full attention to your body's movements. Alternately, find a physical activity that you are unfamiliar with—say, learn a new dance or take a yoga class—and as you're learning new, awkward-feeling moves, take a moment to bring your attention to these unfamiliar physical sensations. If you are not physically active, carve out some time during your day to walk or stretch or swim. When you are engaged in the activity you choose, focus your awareness on your body and movements. If you are walking, for example, pay attention to your steps—how the ground feels under your feet, how your muscles feel when moving.

LISTEN: When you are engaged in a conversation with another person, practice intentional curiosity. Take the time to focus your attention on what your companion is saying and respond only with relevant questions or with acknowledgment that you have heard—put your own input and desire to express opinions on the back burner (remember motivational enhancement?). This is especially powerful when you converse with a child and focus on his or her mind and world. Do you notice any discomfort in forcing yourself to listen? If so, can you describe what that feels like? How does it feel to keep your opinions to yourself? Why do you think you experience this discomfort?

HOW DO OTHERS SEE YOU?: Choose three people in your life. They don't all have to be close to you. You might choose your spouse, a close friend, your boss or employees, your neighbor, your roommate, your mother. In your Personal Journal, compose a picture of yourself through each of their eyes. Do you believe they see you accurately? Do different facets of your character present themselves depending on whom you're with? Keep in mind that this is fine: It's usual that you treat different people differently—like your spouse and your parent. If, for instance, you find yourself patient with one person but short and irritated with another, remember that these are simply facets of yourself. You are not being dishonest or fake just because you behave differently with different people. Self-acceptance (Chapter 5) is key here. On the other hand, when you bring this difference into mindful self-awareness, you might ask whether you want it to persist. *Should* you be as patient with one person with whom you are short-tempered as another with whom you display greater tolerance? This is a trait you obviously are capable of expressing—should you use it more readily?

WHAT ARE YOUR STRENGTHS AND VULNERABILITIES? In your journal, make a list of the areas of your life in which you excel or have excelled in the past. Then make a list of areas of your life where you feel vulnerable. If you have trouble making this list, ask for help from someone you trust. In fact, even if you don't have trouble, you might benefit from doing this exercise with someone you trust. They may provide a more realistic, objective perspective on your answers. If you choose to do this exercise with a companion, note the areas of disagreement.

Shoving Off

The overarching goal of The PERFECT Program is to reach the point where you can lift your sails, free from addiction, and embark on your real life's journey. The skills you have been learning will help you achieve the balance necessary to head off into the sunset, rather than to keep you moored to a program, a label, or a prescribed way of life—whether that be "addiction" or "recovery." It's time to take that step, like the tightrope walker Philippe Petit, depicted in the film *Man on Wire*, taking his first step onto the wire spanning the two World Trade Center towers. (Well, your step is not *quite* that daring.) After all the work you have done, it's time to put what you've learned into play. Let's start by navigating out of the rocky, sometimes perilous port you've been anchored in.

You have identified a vision for your life and have defined some goals—it's time to take some decisive steps, make some real moves. In the previous chapters, you gathered and organized everything that is important to you, the things that bring value, purpose, and meaning to your life, and you made some decisions about where you need some life-management support and skills training. Now, you can bring these elements into present actions. You have thought about life changes you want to make: some monumental or frightening, like leaving a relationship or tackling your debts, and some more gentle and exciting, like starting a garden or going back to college. Regardless of whether your current goals are difficult or simple to activate, getting started—taking that first step off your secure mooring—can be daunting.

We have a tendency to think there is some magic moment in the future when we will be the person we think we should be. Everything must be right in some mystical, undefined way before we can fully exist, as if a square on the calendar held some transformative power: We'll start on Monday. We'll wait until after the holidays. We will wake up a completely different person on New Year's Day. Of course, it can be helpful to pick a date to start making significant changes or to create a new project. If you find that works for you, by all means, get out your calendar and mark it off. At the same time, there is nothing stopping you from making smaller corrections to your course, based on the goals you have set for yourself, this day—this hour. You are here, now, and you can start right where you stand.

Begin by deciding and committing to what is immediately doable and essential—that is, what you can and want to introduce into your life *today*—and beginning to do so. (Exercising regularly, for instance, or doing yoga or meditating.) Next, you will focus on your long-term goals and what you need to do to achieve them. (Going to school, acquiring a new skill, forging intimate relationships with family members, friends, or people as yet unknown.) Finally, you will approach the monumental life changes you want to make and decide on some strategies for setting these in motion. (Moving, forming a partnership, getting divorced, having a child, changing careers.)

You have identified important goals you want to pursue and have decided how you want to approach overcoming your addiction in a way that works for you, based on your values and preferences and your exposure to the ways people overcome addiction, as described in Chapter 2 and throughout this book. Now let's prioritize your necessary steps, starting with things to be addressed immediately—including, of course, your addiction. You may also need to deal quickly with concerns around your family, health, or work. One way to decide what to do now is to address the things that will create chaos if you wait any longer.

You may also want to start to do simple things that will enhance your quality of life—like keeping your residence clean and organized. Think of those things also that you'd like to adopt into your life, like exercise or other wholesome activities. In terms of larger goals, consider your education, career, and perhaps social and family life. And, finally, you may have some serious changes to make to your living situation that may require you to shore up your resources (both financial and emotional), to seek legal counsel, or to venture into territory that is overwhelmingly unfamiliar, such as striking out on your own for the first time. Use your Goals Worksheets to help guide you.

IMMEDIATE: In your PERFECT Journal, list the changes you intend to make now and describe the consequences for you if you do not. Consider how you will implement these changes—break them down into smaller steps and prioritize them. Then make a commitment to yourself by scheduling these things on your calendar. For instance, if you must see a dentist because you are in pain, commit to a time to make the phone call and set the appointment. Similarly, if you plan to go cold turkey on your addiction, commit to it on your calendar. If you are delinquent on your bills and risk being shut off or going to collections, contact your creditors. Get started now, and keep close track of whatever you do to further your goals. Do not forget to make note of how it makes you feel to tick these tasks off your list. If you find yourself overwhelmed by the number of tasks you have set for yourself, go back and reprioritize.

INTERMEDIATE: List in your PERFECT Journal those things you want to bring into your life, and begin setting a sensible schedule for implementing them. You may need to do some research to accomplish this. If so, schedule time for that work. As you did with your immediate plans, make commitments, follow through, and check off their accomplishment. Keep track of your activities and how it makes you feel to pursue these things. In your Personal Journal, if you find that you have lost interest, or that something you have included on your list doesn't live up to your expectations, explore those feelings and ask yourself whether your plans were true to you, why you were wrong in thinking they were, or if there is another reason you have abandoned them.

MAJOR CHANGES: If you are experiencing impending or current major upheavals in your life, you may have a lot of planning to do and hard decisions to make. It could be that making a major change is imperative; it must take top priority and so also becomes an immediate need, albeit a potentially life-altering one. If you are in an abusive or destructive domestic situation or, say, your house is in foreclosure or you are in a serious legal bind, you must focus on this right away. In this case, you may need to find some community, therapeutic, or governmental resources to help you take control of your situation and prioritize the tasks required in order to make changes—or simply to cope with your situation. Use your goal-setting tools and begin taking the steps you need to take to see this through. Chapter 10, about triaging, provides you with lists of resources for difficult or unfamiliar situations.

If the major changes you'd like to make are less emergent—say, a long-coming divorce or a residential move, buying a house, having a child—you can begin to prepare yourself in less dramatic ways. Meanwhile, focus steadily on your addiction and wellness goals so that you are in a stronger position to navigate the inevitable frustrations and surprises that come with tackling your major life goals—put simply, you can't have children or launch a new career while getting drunk daily or having other unaddressed psychological and health issues.

Getting Straight

In the early stages of leaving an addiction, you may have a lot to put in order—many things to remedy and take care of—before you can feel fairly secure in your recovery. The most prominent single finding from Baumeister's research on willpower[1] is that you develop that muscle—become capable of self-regulation—the more you practice it throughout your life.

Honoring your commitments

You may have to clear up quite a bit of baggage and debris following your emergence from addiction. After dropping a lot of balls and sacrificing much to your addiction, correcting your course is not about making up to particular individuals (see Chapter 5, on forgiveness), but about establishing yourself as a worthwhile, dependable person. Doing what you say you're going to do creates a secure identity, both in your mind and the minds of others, and a feeling of having a firm place in your community and the world. Part of making and keeping legitimate commitments is being able to recognize when you are over-committing or making promises that you simply cannot keep just to maintain some peace in the moment or to make someone feel good. If you generally have trouble following through on your promises, here are a couple of approaches to enhancing this skill and value:

- Don't make commitments impulsively, even if someone is pressing you for an answer or it sounds like fun. Take the time to see whether it will fit into your schedule, whether it is something you find important, or whether it will compromise other, more important commitments you have made.
- Practice making and keeping commitments in small ways. Start by, say, scheduling a task and doing it during the time you set for yourself. Find an event that interests you and commit yourself to attending.

Honoring your commitments to yourself is a major value to cultivate—an essential element of mindfulness, self-knowledge, and overall fulfillment.

Domestic space

Moving from your existential place in the world to the most physical space you occupy, having a living space that provides comfort and sanctuary will contribute greatly to your peace of mind. You must decide for yourself what that looks and feels like for you. That might entail putting your kitchen in order so that you can cook meals, or it might mean decluttering your entryway. You might like to have a home that could be featured in *Better Homes and Gardens*, but a more realistic and satisfying target for you may be to avoid a pile of dishes or food rotting in your sink and to sleep on clean sheets. You may be someone who can't rest unless everything is in its place, or you may find that puttering around your house each morning completing small household tasks is calming. Whatever your inclination, start following through on it. Your Goals Worksheet enables you to identify key areas to focus on—begin there. Here are some ideas and resources that may help you get going:

Getting help and exploring resources: You may be in a position to hire a home organization expert or a cleaning service to come in and do a deep clean. Don't be reluctant to do so because you're embarrassed by whatever mess you have. They've seen it all. (Which I, as an addiction therapist, might also say—in case you need to consult someone like me.) You can also enlist a good friend to come in and help (as described in Chapter 7). Another option is to seek out a local co-op group, or start one yourself, of people who all meet at one member's house on the weekend and work together to tackle the domestic chores.

Accountability: Free online resources can provide you with accountability and direction. Here are some websites that you might find useful: Flylady.net is a coaching resource that helps you prioritize your household tasks. Rememberthemilk.com is a task manager, which you can use online or as an app for your phone. Do some exploring; see if you can find other resources with a built-in community of people who are working toward the same goal.

Social Skills: Creating Community and Intimacy

Community

Our communities consist of our families, living mates, neighbors, social networks, co-workers, activity partners, church congregations, towns and cities. Nothing enhances our sense of purpose, of belonging on earth, of meaning, of contentment more than does feeling part of a community. This is fundamental to the human condition, and the general loss of community in modern culture is a severe blow to all our humanity—as well as being a major cause of addiction. Addicted people tend to form pseudo-communities around their addictions (think again of Rose in Chapter 1), and often their fear of losing that pseudo-community is a strong component in maintaining an addiction. That is, people fear they will be lonely if they are deprived of their addiction mates. Conversely, forming positive communities is a strong antidote to addiction and is even used as a form of treatment, social network therapy, as described in Chapter 7. Reconnecting with such non-addiction-focused, real-world groups in meaningful ways will bring you a deeper and more satisfying sense of belonging than addiction ever can.

EXERCISE: In your journal, compose a list of the communities you are involved in or touch upon. Acknowledge your connections to the world.

Make another list of some others you would like to be part of. Depending on your personality, you may want to limit yourself pretty much to family or a close social circle, and your neighborhood; or you may want to involve yourself in a number of different areas involving special interests you have or want to pursue. Imagine how you would participate in these groups, and then ask yourself if it is realistic to make the commitment. Complete a Goals Worksheet to help you prioritize and decide what steps to take to find and join such communities.

Making friends

Joining communities has much in common with making friends—finding compatible and accessible people with whom to spend time, share interests, and perhaps develop deeper feelings and relationships—up to and including love. People—as we discussed in the last chapter—have different degrees of sociability, of skill at and tolerance for interacting with others, of enjoying time alone. But it's fair to say that everybody needs some degree of skill at both being alone and being with others. A free life can't be lived without some version of both traits. If you can never be alone, then you can never be at ease and must always desperately seek out contact—for better or for worse (see the case below). If you can't spend some time with and interact with people, then you can be shut into yourself—sentenced to aloneness that is a kind of addiction.

The short answer to how to be able to live both parts of yourself is—as with nearly everything in this book—practice. Schedule time to spend by yourself—something you must, of course, do when you are meditating. Reading, listening to music, walking, being with a pet—all of those do count (the PERFECT Program is very open-minded). Watching television counts if you do it purposefully, because you are specifically watching something you enjoy for reasons you know. And schedule time to interact with others. This may mean going to one of the groups you described in the previous section. Or it may mean calling and speaking with, or arranging to visit or meet, an old friend, a relation, or someone you'd like to get to know—for any reason whatsoever. It is a mark of our times—and it is not a good mark—that actual contact with people, even so much as talking by phone, is becoming a relic of the past. Nothing against e-mails and iPads, but we can't do without human contact.

CASE: Isaac had been a good student. But when he arrived at his large, well-regarded high school, he suddenly seemed intimidated. And so, for most of his first semester, he walked around the school as though he were in a penitentiary. Of course, Isaac's parents—Rachel and Bob—were worried. And, so, when he returned home one day with a smile and said he had lunch with a few kids, one of whom he liked especially, his parents were glad.

But it turned out that this outsider's group was heavily immersed in drugs. Thus followed four years of hell for Isaac's parents, ending when they used a large part of their life savings to send Isaac to a residential treatment program. The program seemed like a good one, although Rachel and Bob questioned some aspects of it. Was it really true that Isaac had inherited a disease and that he could never drink (let alone take drugs) for the rest of his life? After all, he was only nineteen. Moreover, when he graduated the three-month program, he was sent to a residence. But in many ways the kids in this group were a lot like those he was with in high school, only now supposedly recovering.

But what most worried Rachel and Bob was that, as they kept up with the parents of the other kids they met in treatment and the group home, nearly all of their children had relapsed. How is that possible, Bob asked Rachel, after they learned so much and did so well interacting with one another in treatment and the halfway house? What had occurred, of course, is that they had simply fit in again with their substance-abusing peer groups as soon as they returned home.

The crucial issue at every point in Isaac's story is how easily he formed relationships, with whom he did so, and in what direction the friends he made pulled him. Isaac's story is about the centrality of friendship formation and dealing with others in addiction and recovery. Learning social skills like those in the previous chapter in order to meet diverse and healthy individuals is an essential element of an addiction-free life.

Intimacy, love, and addiction

Love is one of those large goals that an awful lot of people pursue—and that an awful lot attain in one or more forms (including spouses, friends, and children). But it's no sure thing, and—depending on how far you are starting behind in your life—it may take you some time to acquire and assemble these resources. They then become the building blocks outlined in this chapter and the rest of *Recover!* for forming truly satisfying relationships. This is because love—as Archie Brodsky and I indicated in *Love and Addiction*—is built on the exact opposite foundation from an addiction. Addiction stems from the absence of connections to life and substitutes for such connections. Love flourishes best when you have the *most* points of contact with the world, including other positive relationships. Addictive love relationships are most likely when you are desperately seeking emotional sustenance from other people while you haven't yet created the necessary basis for sharing such intense feelings by having a solid life in place.

Practical Skills: Education, Work, Financial

Education and work

Don't assume that you have ruined the connections you have to every part of your life and every person in it because of your addiction. You may have hurt them but, often, many can still be rescued. I have offered several case studies of people who are successful at their jobs despite their addiction (of course, other areas of their lives suffer). So don't reject—in anticipation of being rejected—any parts of your life that have survived your addiction even as you work to improve them. For example, if you haven't been fired, don't quit your job out of guilt.

However, for many, keeping a job or pursuing an education has fallen by the wayside. If you're in that category, you may be wondering where to start—and completing your Goals Worksheet leaves you feeling lost. How do you set realistic goals for yourself when you feel so far behind or so far out of your element that you can't even be sure what your real options are? Do you know how to look for and apply for a job, what courses to take at school, how you will pay for these courses, or what degree suits you best?

CASE: Thomas had been smoking pot regularly for so long that all he could do was sell the drug to others as a way of getting by. He had once been a quite capable computer programmer. But he was long past the point of feeling up-to-date with writing code, the Internet, and information technology skills. Whenever he considered quitting smoking grass, he was confronted with the enormity of the barriers separating him from the real work world. How could he *begin* to reengage?

Of course, Thomas had once been able to obtain jobs in information technology. As always, getting started—or restarted—is intimidating. You may imagine the barriers as higher than they are. In any case, there is no alternative other than to begin. Thomas began taking online courses, which are readily available and accessible. As he settled into doing course exercises, he saw that his old skills were still relevant; he even compared favorably with others taking the courses, according to the published grade curves. In a short time, he was applying for jobs (albeit having to fashion crafty explanations for the gaps in his resume—fortunately, he had never been arrested). The process wasn't dramatic, and Thomas wasn't where he would have been if he hadn't devoted several years to his drug of choice. But, then, life is a process, always beginning with now.

For specific practical suggestions for continuing or resuming your education, getting a better job, or starting a business, see Chapter 10, "Triage."

Financial

Money management can be enormously stressful, especially for those in the throes of an addiction who have allowed bills to pile up or who are avoiding calls from creditors or the IRS. Addictions are expensive habits that lead you to spend money you don't have—especially if your addiction is gambling or shopping. Of course, the cost of liquor or cigarettes or street drugs also adds up, as does that for virtually every addiction. You may know about waking up in a panic over money in the middle of the night.

But no matter how painful it is to contemplate, this is an area you simply must get under control, because it will weigh you down until you do. Dealing with finances can be an unappetizing task if you are in debt or behind on your bills. As anxious as dealing with your finances makes you, however, worrying about your money when you don't have a handle on it is far worse. It is imperative that you know where your ground zero is. In this as in other areas of your life, you are able to address and fix only what you are able to see clearly.

So let's tackle finances and restore your peace of mind. Whatever the mess you have on your hands involves, you can pull yourself out of it and keep yourself out. Schedule time on your calendar to devote to this. When that time comes, shut off your phone, iPad, and so on, and then break this task down into a series of manageable mini-goals such as those outlined in Chapter 10, "Triage." It's possible that you will have to explore bankruptcy. That's a big topic for which this book is not the right source of advice. But be aware of it as a possibility.

Personal Skills: Your Health and Well-Being

Self-care

Since addiction can cause you to disregard so many aspects of your life, your ability to care for yourself diligently may also have suffered. Personal hygiene is not just something you do to make yourself presentable to the world; it is something you do for you. Showering and brushing your teeth regularly, sleeping and eating well, getting dressed every morning, exercising, visiting the doctor, washing your clothes—all are absolutely important. First, they foster a sense of self-respect and energy and help you develop wholesome habits. They engage you in acts of self-nurturance, which you deserve. They signal that you are ready to participate in your own life. If you have slacked off on your self-care practices, ask yourself how, and begin bringing these good habits back into your life.

Leisure pursuits

Since addiction takes up so much time and energy, you may have some time on your hands. Boredom, restlessness, aimlessness, and obsessive, intrusive thoughts can be powerful instigators of relapse, and not knowing what to do with yourself can be emotionally and morally excruciating. Do you remember a time in your life—most likely in your childhood—when you could lose yourself in play and creativity? Perhaps you—alone or with friends—were able to invent an elaborate pretend world, characters, and scenarios that kept you engrossed all day long! Recapturing this part of your life—your creativity and sense of pure, free fun—is as important to your life as it is for you to start bringing order to the chaos. When you have such a sense of joy, everything—reading, walking and hiking, seeing people, being alone—can open up to you. Pull out your Goals Worksheet and fill it in with activities that will spark your interests, sense of play, and feelings of accomplishment. You might include art, volunteering, spending time with your children or grandchildren, cooking, exercising, learning a new skill, taking a class, and on and on.

Spiritual or humanitarian

If you practice a particular belief system or religion, or if you honor your place in the grand scheme of things as a member of the human race, consider giving your spiritual or belief system or humanitarian impulses a bigger place in your life. This investment will contribute greatly to your sense of purpose and community, infusing your life and actions with meaning. You may seek out a congregation that feels like a good fit for you, join a meditation group, or volunteer for a cause that you support, with the intention of building community around this important area of your life. Doing so—especially if you lack family or community support—will broaden your scope and give you a comforting sense of your place in the world.

Mental health

As you begin to drill down into the areas of your life that need attention, you may become aware of underlying mental health issues. Perhaps you have already been diagnosed as having—or believe that you may have—bipolar disorder, anxiety, depression, post-traumatic stress disorder, or some other type of psychiatric condition or disorder. Not to minimize these disorders, it is safe to say that we all have some experience of them and other emotional conditions and trauma. As I described in Chapter 2 on addiction and recovery, emotional problems are both causes of and responses to addiction, while at the same time they are important issues for recovery. The good news is that many of the techniques and practices you are learning in The PERFECT Program are equally useful for combating these emotional problems or disorders. So, feelings that you've been masking with addiction may emerge in full force, but you are also developing positive and powerful ways of coping with them.

However, just as with the case of seeking bankruptcy relief, there are matters that go beyond the scope of *Recover!*'s aims. If you need help with serious emotional problems that haunt your ability not only to escape addiction, but also to live fruitfully, you should seek professional help. My approach is obviously consistent with cognitive-behavioral therapy (CBT) and pragmatically oriented counseling, and so I favor that type of treatment. In America today, it is hard to find such help in psychiatry, which is dominated by pharmaceutical treatments. *Recover!* and The PERFECT Program don't generally go well with drug treatments, although they don't rule them out or disparage them—as long as the medications are combined with counseling. Of course, the quality of the counseling remains a critical issue, and receiving good—or even safe—treatment is by no means guaranteed. In HMOs and other institutional care settings, the psychiatrist prescribes drugs while a psychologist or social worker provides CBT or supportive therapy. Sometimes—too often—supportive therapy simply permits venting that enables people's complaining and blaming others. Psychiatrists, meanwhile, are becoming less able—both by training and due to economic constraints—to practice any kind of psychotherapy.

Where therapy is provided—whether by a psychologist, social worker, or other trained counselor or, occasionally, a psychiatrist—the favored type is now CBT on the grounds that it addresses your problems directly and has been shown to be effective. Psychoanalytically oriented ("talk") therapy, on the other hand, is increasingly difficult to find or be reimbursed for. Feel free to explain what your perspective is and what you seek in exploring and entering any type of mental health relationship.[2] And there is no way for you to eliminate your own critical decision making in deciding whether your therapy is being helpful.

Reframing Failure

Once you start taking deliberate steps to make things happen in your life and develop healthier habits of mind and action, you will certainly find yourself missing the mark on some of the goals you have set for yourself. In times like this, you might recall Woody Allen's famous dictum: "Ninety percent of life is just showing up." To put this in the context of The PERFECT Program: "showing up" means that your conscious presence and awareness *is* your success. Your engaged participation is all that's required, even if the results don't always measure up. You are now using the skills you've learned in the task of making broad and permanent changes in your life. But the key changes cannot be measured by how flawlessly you succeed at the things you set out to do. What's important is that you *made the decision* to do them and *pursued your goals mindfully*—that is, intentionally, investing yourself in the process and keeping track of the results. What you're now doing is living your life.

Incorporating the essential elements of your true self into your life is an exercise of your free will, which may have wilted from neglect. You are training your true self to take over for your addicted self, which will, ultimately, make addiction irrelevant. Developing any weak muscle can be painful and make you hyper-aware of the strength of your addiction. Imagine, for example, trying to write clearly and automatically with your non-dominant, or "wrong," hand. The resulting awkwardness and sloppiness shout out to you that you could so easily switch back and just get it over with, resorting to the muscles (or habits) you relied on before. Embarking on your recovery process will bring similar moments of awkwardness and distress. You will feel tempted to resume familiar but destructive habits when you fail at your new efforts. Whether you do or you don't, you may judge yourself harshly. This self-punishment may feel correct, but ultimately it blocks your forward motion.

For example, say that one of your modest changes was to bring a new plant into your house, to give your environment a sense of vibrancy. But then your plant died because you didn't water or fertilize it properly. Your reaction might be brutal self-recrimination: "I am such a loser; I can't even keep a plant alive. What's wrong with me?!" But it's just going to happen sometimes that your best intentions won't pan out. While recognizing this, you needn't allow yourself to accept failure. Plan for failure and learn to reframe it with compassion: *This is not failure; it's information.* You'll do better the next time. Either that, or you're just not a plant person.

When you reframe failure as information (or feedback), you maintain your sense of active engagement, control, and forward movement. If you walk into the gym for the first time and try to match the resistance the last person set on a machine, you probably will be unable to lift it. This could be embarrassing if anyone were looking (although no one is), but in any case it's not the end of the world. You don't leave the gym or give up or throw a tantrum (now *that* people would notice). You simply get real about your abilities, adjust the weights accordingly, rest a bit, and then begin to become stronger gradually and sensibly. Similarly, if you make an attempt at something life-affirming and find that you are unable to see it through, take the opportunity to gather information about your blind spots and your unreal expectations. But always remain mindful of the purpose behind your attempt.

EXERCISE: In your Personal Journal, think of a recent failure and write about it: What were you trying to accomplish? What went wrong? What do you think this says about you? Now, try to look at the scenario more objectively and compassionately: Were you trying to do something that requires habits not yet in your repertoire? Were you attempting to take on more responsibility than you could reasonably handle or fit into your schedule? Did you start at a place that turned out to be over your depth? Were there steps you missed? Situations you avoided? If so, why? If you were allowed a do-over, would you try this again? If not, why not? And if so, what would you do differently?

Detour: Relapse!

Speaking of reframing failure, the subject of relapse is surely on your mind. It is not inevitable, but it happens. You can prepare for it both by anticipating and avoiding it and by developing techniques for righting your course after it happens. Relapse is a return to addictive behavior—a backslide—which occurs after a period of progress. The impact of relapse can be very demoralizing, making you feel as if you were back at square one, or a hopeless case. What causes it? How does it happen and why?

Alan Marlatt began his research on relapse prevention by investigating what caused smokers, alcoholics, and heroin addicts to relapse.[3] The standard interpretations were that (1) their withdrawal symptoms simply overcame them, or (2) in a conditioned response, people were exposed to stimuli associated with their former use, and this association created irresistible cravings to use.[4] But when Marlatt actually questioned addicts, he found that they were unlikely to relapse when experiencing intense physical urges to use, as occur during the immediate withdrawal period. Rather, relapses were responses to negative emotions and conflicts that the study subjects previously may have used their addiction to address and that exceeded their abilities to manage without their addiction. Or else they relapsed when they entered a setting where they had used or were with people they had used with before.

Based on these findings, Marlatt developed relapse prevention techniques to supplement environmental planning—that is, staying away from "bad" places, people, and things. Relapse prevention focuses on people's coping mechanisms for dealing with stress (or even pleasure) in general, and specifically for addressing cravings to use that appear either randomly or in challenging emotional situations. Himself a longtime practitioner of meditation (to which he credited his remission from hypertension), Marlatt was moved to see whether and how meditation could be part of the cornucopia of techniques for combating relapse, including cravings. The results led in the direction we have picked up from Marlatt and other researchers and adapted and expanded for The PERFECT Program.[5] Marlatt's work has always had a sound scientific basis. The value added through The PERFECT Program is to develop and tailor these techniques in ways that are personally and clinically useful, since Alan himself never wrote any popular guides for people to follow.

Simply put, a relapse is triggered by imbalance. The situation at hand or the triggering event overwhelms your ability to cope while you are developing new skills, resources, and perspectives. Recalling the "dominant hand" analogy, in which your dominant hand represents your ingrained habits, imagine that you are diligently practicing handling all your daily tasks with your weaker hand. Despite the awkwardness, you are becoming more adept all the time. But one day, without warning, someone pitches a ball directly at your head. You instinctively reach out to grab the ball with your dominant hand.* That is just about how relapse works, and there are several scenarios and life events that might trigger it:

*All analogies are inexact, and the "handedness" example is so because, unlike addiction, handedness, in most cases, is largely determined in the brain and is inborn. This example has the added disadvantage that there is a history of bias against left-handers that has sometimes taken the form of forcing them to use their right hand (I write with my left hand). The ball-catching example is the better example of learned handedness than writing, since most kids learn to catch best with the hand on which they wear their glove—the opposite hand from the one with which they throw a ball, not because that hand is especially adept at catching.

- Stressful situations
- Major or milestone events
- Strong emotions, including anger and even joy
- Unexpectedly powerful triggers that seem to arise out of the blue
- Loneliness, boredom, anxiety, restlessness, hopelessness, or any other painful or difficult feelings
- Being around people who undermine your goals
- Romanticized memories of the benefits of using, while forgetting or downplaying the consequences
- Unaddressed mental health concerns, such as depression, that require attention.

Can you think of other relapse triggers?

EXERCISE: In your PERFECT Journal, in the "Triggers" section (page 155), write down any situations that might trigger a relapse—or that have in the past. Can you identify exactly how your skills, resources, and perspective were outmatched by the situation? What action could you have taken to prevent the relapse? Or what could you have done/do to get yourself back on track?

Reframing relapse

As in our discussion of failure, a relapse can provide you with a wealth of information you can use to continue down your path to wellness. If you experience a relapse, use it as an opportunity to increase your self-knowledge. Make note of everything that led up to it: your life circumstances, the triggers you experienced, the self-deception that you now recognize. You should ask yourself how you can avoid or improve the circumstances leading to relapse, or whether you ignored feelings welling up in you that signaled where you were heading. Did your decision to indulge make you feel as if you were doing something good for yourself, like loosening a noose around your neck? What benefit, exactly, were you seeking? What in your life represents the noose? Are there parts of your life that you have been ignoring while seeking to improve other areas? If so, what changes can you make in your situation that will relieve some of the burden you feel?

You are now engaged in truth seeking about your addiction—where, when, and why it arises. Do your best to discover the truth. This is actually step one of mindfulness practice, recognizing and responding to cravings and other urges to resort to addictive behavior. If you have not yet been able to incorporate your mindfulness practice into your daily schedule, now is the time to make it a priority. Turn back to Chapter 4 to review your meditation and other techniques. This is a skill that will serve you enormously in relapse prevention, because it allows you to recognize and to ride out—or to recuperate from—uncomfortable feelings, like cravings, with the knowledge that they will pass. The practice of mindfulness will also expand your horizons, allowing you to identify the range of your options. Where before you might not have realized you had any choices, you now know there are a host of responses to insert between your urges and your addiction. Finally, continuing to exercise mindfulness in relapse prevention develops your ability to turn your attention where you choose to, away from triggers.

The central concept to keep in mind where relapse is concerned is that it is not failure. This means that, if you relapse, you aren't "starting over." In fact, "starting over" has no real meaning. Twelve-step programs make a virtue of "time." Members count their days—even hours and minutes—of "sobriety." They require people to start their count over if they have a relapse. So, if you have been "sober" for five years and then have a beer one day, you're back at day one. I would say this was silly if it weren't so destructive. Please recall my discussion of "hitting bottom" in Chapter 4. Go beyond this superstitious, irrational way of thinking, one that has created such ineffective approaches to recovery.

Getting back on track

Believing that you have completely and irreparably botched recovery is an example of the all-or-nothing perfectionist thinking that underlies addiction. It is clearly lacking in self-compassion. You always, always have the option to gather yourself and continue on your path. This is as open to you as—in fact, it is more common than—the AA-endorsed view that you have to throw in the towel. Even considering the latter as a possibility is wrong. At this point, you have the understanding, skills, resources, and perspective to make a conscious decision to continue on your path with mindfulness and self-regard. Remember Renee from Chapter 3, who, after six years' abstinence from alcohol, went into a bar, drank, got intoxicated, drove drunk, and lost her license, her job, and her husband? All of that was unnecessary. Even so, she quickly righted herself and didn't return to a life of drinking. By that point, recovery remained for her—despite her bad decisions and choices—the most relevant, easily accessed option in life.

Exercise: Relapse Moments of Truth

At times, you may be tempted to return to your addiction, when you have cravings—even compulsions—to use, say, when you are in an environment where you previously used, when you are vulnerable emotionally, when life has thrown you a number of challenges and defeats, or even sometimes triumphs and successes! How you deal with these moments determines your ability to navigate your recovery. Answer these questions in your PERFECT Journal:

1. Describe three situations in which you are most likely to use.
2. Visualize each situation and describe your feelings in it.
3. Describe a strategy for each that you can rely on instead of using.
4. Who would you call if you were thinking about using but wanted to resist? Why?
5. Who would you call if you had been using but wanted to avoid further damage? Why?

Should you discuss these roles with those individuals right away?

I have emphasized the idea that every moment is an opportunity to make a good decision. In other words, just because you have taken a single step in the direction of a steep cliff, it doesn't mean that you are now required to take a running leap off the edge. This image opposes the 12-step or hijacked-brain notion that your misstep has propelled you off the cliff and your relapse is, like gravity, an irresistible force of nature. Relapsing after using is not like gravity. Your mindfulness skills will help you identify your moments of grace and give you the presence of mind to act on them at any point after the moment you veer off course so as to realign yourself with your values.

CASE: Martha, who has been battling an addiction to prescription painkillers, has recently decided to go cold turkey. She's had some difficult moments, but has been able to stay on track by keeping her focus on creating order out of chaos. That has brought her a great sense of fulfillment and peace of mind. One day, as she was in the middle of cleaning a hallway closet that she had been using to stow all sorts of unusable junk, she was overcome by a seemingly random urge to stop what she was doing and visit a friend of hers who kept a well-stocked pharmacy in her pocketbook. Almost as soon as the thought crossed her mind, Martha jumped up and called her friend ("I'm so sick of sorting all this junk! I've been good for a month already!"), who was more than happy to accommodate her. Martha threw on a pair of jeans, drove to her friend's house, plunked herself down on the couch, and swallowed the pills offered to her with a freshly opened beer. (Remember that, besides this being a relapse, it is also always dangerous to combine painkillers with other drugs or alcohol.) The two of them spent the night watching reality shows and giggling senselessly, and everything seemed to fall back into place.

The next morning, Martha woke up feeling terrible—and the self-recrimination was worse than the hangover.

What happened? At what point did Martha lose her perspective? It was as if a tornado picked her up out of the blue, right out of the messy closet, and plunked her down on her friend's couch with a couple of pills in one hand and a beer in the other. And what now? How does she handle the cravings and old habits?

What happened? Martha's "dominant hand" simply asserted itself and began to function on auto-pilot, as it will do. Habits, well-established patterns of thought and behavior, can take over in moments of vulnerability—this cannot be avoided all the time. Remember that as you progress, these moments will become fewer and farther between. But you may encounter them quite often at the outset. The key is not to pretend that you can—or should—evade them every time, but to recognize that you're off course and take steps to correct.

Consider how many opportunities Martha has to avoid full-blown relapse and to realign her actions with her values. Perhaps, at this early stage in her journey, she wasn't able to correct course as soon as she would have liked to. Blindsided by an urge whose momentum she couldn't fight, she ended up on a trajectory that led her to a familiar, painful place. She may remember that this overwhelming urge hit her when she was sorting through some items that brought back painful memories or reminded her of a time when she was enjoying the situations that led to her addiction. Or, perhaps, she was overcome by the tedium of the task, or she was

FIGURE 8.1

Navigating Relapse

At any time, before or after you veer off your course, you can tack back to your true path by using the skills, practices, knowledge, and exercises you have learned through The PERFECT Program.
No matter how far off you go, there is always a way back.

The PERFECT Program tacks back to your true course.

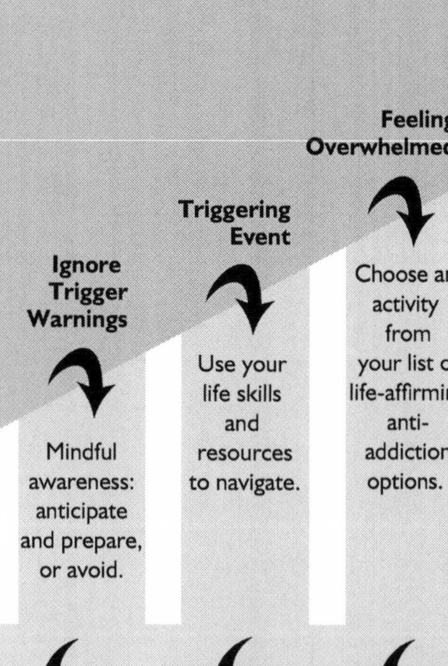

berating herself for letting things get so out of control. Or, perhaps, she was even thinking how great she was doing in her new life!

At the moment she wakes up, overcome with regret, she has a choice: to give up on herself or to forgive herself, take an honest look at what happened, and make some decisions. There is always a window of opportunity, allowing you to correct course, no matter how far down the wrong path you have gone, as Figure 8.1 shows.

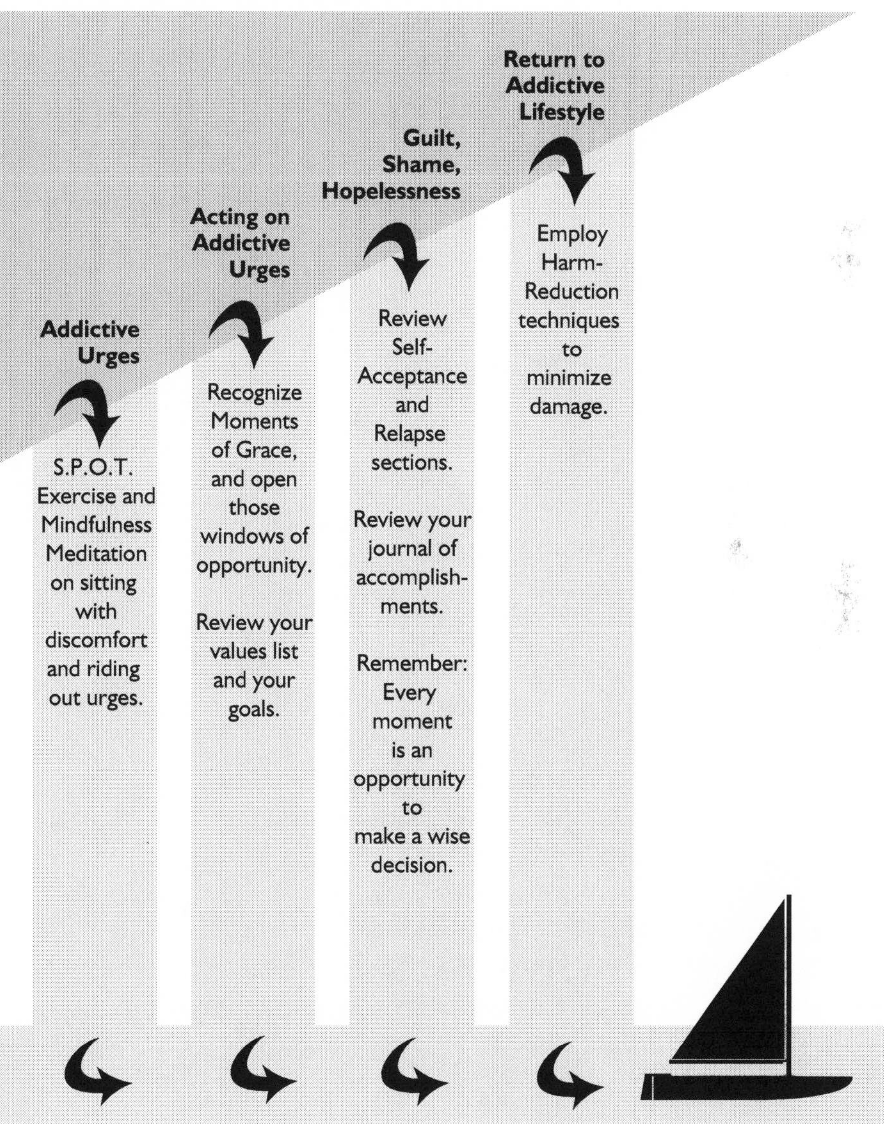

Remember these things about relapse:

- Relapse is not failure; it's information.
- Relapse does not mean starting over from scratch.
- Relapse does not mean that you will never recover.
- Relapse can be reversed at any stage—you do not have to pursue it to "rock bottom."

You have the skills to realign yourself and continue with your recovery.

Avoiding relapse for love, eating, and other non-abstinent addictions

Some activities that some people find addictive, as I discussed in Chapter 3, can never be completely avoided. How can addicts avoid relapse when, in a sense, they have never stopped doing the activity? Think of eating. You will continue to eat on a weight-loss program. You may carefully avoid some foods, maintain your weight, and support weight loss with exercise. But you will not always follow your diet perfectly; no one can, and to attempt perfection—as always—can cause problems, in this case the sister addictions of obesity (i.e., bulimia and anorexia).

And, so, what happens when you as a dieter—say, one who has lost a considerable amount of weight—eats pasta or bread, or a cookie or some other sweet, that you have been rigorously avoiding? Indeed, *how* you handle these events is a mark of the *success* of your recovery. Say you have some pie or pasta. You will want to have a reasonable portion, which you can define differently according to the situation or where you feel you are in your recovery. Being able to eat these foods mindfully,[6] both enjoyably and carefully, provides you with sufficient rewards that you no longer crave them as "forbidden fruits."

At the same time, you—while eating the food—will be mindful that this is the kind of food that has hurt you in the past and that you cannot start indulging in the way you used to. You might surface an image of your former self eating this dish indiscriminately—even imagining yourself at your former weight. And it is summoning such images, with the commitment not to return to the misery, unhealthiness, and fear they inspire, that is the best guarantee that you will limit potential eating binges. Of course, to regain all of a considerable amount of lost weight is the result of more than one—more than several—such episodes. To return to your former weight would require you to altogether abandon your new lifestyle and way of eating, and the rewards your fitness and appearance have given you, in favor of those fleeting rewards provided by sweets, carbohydrates, and other comfort foods and snacks. You just don't relapse in an instant; doing so means that you have reversed the entire recovery journey you have been on for months and years.

Balance

Getting started on your life's journey with a sense of perspective—informed by mindfulness, self-awareness, and compassion; your values, mission, goals, and your skills and resources—is a monumental step. Knowing who you are, where you want to go, what you want to accomplish, how you're going to accomplish it, and how you will stay focused on the path you have created for yourself, while skillfully navigating all the bumps in the road—like failure and relapse—is a lifelong process. It's essentially what life is all about. It's the very foundation of wisdom. To keep moving forward on your journey requires an ability to keep your attention constantly on your path. But it also requires your ability to *return* your attention to your path when you have lost track. Your mindfulness practice will strengthen your ability to return your focus to where it belongs, and your self-acceptance will give you the perspective and balance that allow you to do so.

Moving Forward

Launching your recovery and leaving addiction behind is not a bed of roses—you will encounter troubling moments that expose your vulnerabilities. But the odds favor your moving forward, and this chapter has helped you find the frame of mind—along with the techniques—to make sure this will happen. Balance is key. But maintaining balance requires strength and movement. These will develop as you continue on your path, learning to keep your perspective when things go wrong. You are on your way! Fully experiencing the non-addictive rewards you are finding will make clear your preference for this new life. Your decision to embark on this path is something to acknowledge and focus on; it is sufficiently important that the next chapter is devoted to celebrating your accomplishments, as well as all of the rediscovered facets of your life that bring you satisfaction, meaning, and joy.

CHAPTER 9

Celebrate

Joy—Honoring your accomplishments while living mindfully and meaningfully

CHAPTER GOALS

- To learn to replace the superficial rewards of addiction with genuine fulfillment
- To track your successes
- To honor your accomplishments
- To practice what you value
- To create traditions and reasons to celebrate
- To discover joy

Purpose: If the consequences of addiction weren't so destructive, you wouldn't be on this journey to wellness; but before you ever experienced the consequences, you experienced the rewards of addiction. Yes, rewards. Imagine that every time you took a drink you skipped right over the part where you felt relief, relaxation, and inebriation and were, instead, socked with an instant hangover. You simply wouldn't do it. Through addiction, we learn to expect instant gratification in the form of oblivion and euphoria, among other benefits. These are powerful, but fleeting, experiences. When enmeshed in addiction, however, we don't recognize—let alone experience and revel in—the many rewards we are blessed with daily, just by living mindfully and meaningfully. This recognition is a crucial life skill to develop, because the reason you are making this journey is to move *from* addiction and *into* fulfillment. And reaping the rewards of your efforts is what it's all about! Learning to replace the superficial, indeed infantile, rewards of addiction with the deep and abiding joys of freedom is the linchpin of your recovery. Doing so will reinforce your sense of momentum and your faith in your abilities, allow you to see how far you have come, and connect you with the joy and satisfaction of living according to your values.

How Far You Have Come

Many of us gloss over our successes and milestones, perhaps believing that it would be unseemly to make a big deal about them or that it would be premature to go counting our chickens before they're hatched. We may feel we don't deserve to recognize achievements that should have been a matter of course all along ("Why should I celebrate cleaning out the fridge—normal people have clean refrigerators and don't throw a party over it") and that we shouldn't start patting ourselves on the back until we can plant our personal flag on the moon. If this describes you (as it does, to some extent, all of us), perhaps it's time to balance your perspective. Making note of your achievements and milestones is not just a trivial self-indulgence. It is a process that, first, ensures that you maintain your non-addictive path forward. Second, knowing how to recognize and celebrate your often hard-won successes is the essence of a joyful life.

In terms of The PERFECT Program, you certainly have come a long way! Let's take a look back at where you have been on this journey and what you have accomplished so far, before you embark on your home stretch. You have, among other things:

- Achieved a realistic understanding of the nature of addiction and recovery
- Gained clarity on how addiction has manifested in your life
- Developed basic mindfulness skills that will support your recovery
- Learned to treat yourself—and others—with compassion
- Rediscovered your priorities: what brings meaning, value, and purpose to your life
- Implemented anti-addiction techniques in your daily life
- Started honing the life skills you need to navigate effectively in the world
- Created a vision for your future
- Set achievable goals in many different areas of your life
- Started taking action to achieve your goals

If you have not had the opportunity to absorb your accomplishments so far, please take a moment now to reflect on this list. And, if you feel you're not where you should be—haven't touched every base—I hope you will reassess your judgment with self-compassion. Remember that while the nature of a book requires that it progress in some logical order, your path out of addiction is uniquely your own. You may have to linger longer than you'd like in different phases of your recovery. It's not a race. And remember, as I mentioned in the last two chapters, you can't avoid obstacles and setbacks, but you can navigate them in a way that's true to yourself and your vision.

PERFECT JOURNAL: Look back over your journey so far and make note of all the things you are proud of and all the steps you have taken, including meaningful shifts in perspective. Forget anything you think should mitigate or negate your sense of accomplishment (say you were abstinent for a month, but had a setback); just focus on every positive step.

Celebrating your successes means taking every opportunity you can to absorb and reinforce the sense of fulfillment you are striving for. Just as there is no sense in waiting to make a positive decision, there's no reason to wait for some arbitrary milestone or ultimate fantasy to materialize before you can begin taking joy and satisfaction from your journey. That doesn't mean you have to take out an announcement in the local paper every time you complete a task. It simply means recognizing and enjoying what you have accomplished—and of course, some accomplishments will warrant a much grander display. Making a habit of honoring yourself and your values—like everything else you have been doing—takes practice, since it may not be your natural impulse.

Tracking Your Progress

One of the most practical ways you can begin creating this new habit of joyous self-appreciation is by tracking your progress daily. I encouraged you to begin this practice in the last chapter because it is a powerful way of keeping yourself focused. At the same time, marking your progress also allows you to see, very concretely, how far you have come and provides the basis for experiencing a sense of pride in your advances. Tracking is an essential practice in that it offers a balanced and objective view of where you are. We often don't recognize how much we are changing; instead, we take our current assets and grace as simply givens, or else miss them entirely. When you look at your chart, you can't deny that you have actually done positive things—it's right there in black and white!

There are many ways to track your progress. You might keep your goals chart next to your bed or on your desk, where you will see it every day. There are computer programs that allow you to do this; you can set such a program to open as soon as you turn on your computer. Many people find the very act of tracking enjoyable. You may get a lot of satisfaction from checking in on a daily basis and entering your facts and figures. Since we are all wired differently, the process might, on the other hand, seem painstaking to you. Don't worry. There are as many ways of tracking as there are people, and you can find the one that jibes best with your personality.

You want to make sure that whatever method you choose is one you will actually use. If you enjoy keeping lists and charts, you may find that a free website like sparkpeople.com is right up your alley. It offers incentives to log on every day and track your goals—whether those are weight-, wellness-, or fitness-related—using an array of online tracking tools, including your own personal blog. But if you would feel overwhelmed by such an energetic and relentless tracking system, you might consider using Jerry Seinfeld's famous "Don't Break the Chain"* approach, which simply requires you to put an *X* on every day that you meet your daily goal, with the intention, eventually, of keeping the chain of *X*s intact. You will be able to see in a quick glance just how many days you stayed on track and take satisfaction in seeing your chain lengthen.

You may also find that a dedicated notebook or calendar works well for you. For example, suppose you want to track your addiction, with the intention of achieving complete abstinence. You might create a simple chart for yourself that you can fill in daily, with headings that are relevant to your goals. For example, see Table 9.1.

You can create your own charts based on whatever addiction-specific goals you are aiming for. Even if you are not meeting your goals on the schedule you have set for yourself, remember to acknowledge your

* At the beginning of each year, Jerry hangs up a "year-at-a-glance" calendar; each day he composes new material he marks with an *X*. This is one way for creative people to impose structure and enforce self-discipline in a lonely form of work.

TABLE 9.1: **Addiction Use Goals**

Date	Did you use today?	Did you want to use today?	What triggered your urges?	Were you able to resist or stop?	If so, why? If not, why?	Strategies	Accomplishments

efforts—which are valuable in themselves—and to focus on your forward momentum. And, as with anything else I have discussed, take account of what works best for you. This isn't an abstract program invented who knows where by who knows whom—it's your life.

Honoring Your Successes

How, exactly, do you honor your successes? What does that mean and what do you do? Say you have made some progress. What do you do about that? I'm not going to present a self-congratulations chart. But what you do and think is measured against the criterion that it enriches your life—including the idea of "joy." Your journey is not about putting your head down and forging on like a martyr until you arrive at a certain destination, upon which you can finally put your feet up and relax. There is no such place. The sun always comes up; you always have challenges to meet, milestones to celebrate, and places to go. Fulfillment is not the end of the road. It is the road.

Say, for instance, that one of your goals is to lose a significant amount of weight (something I have done). You embark on a plan that really works well for you: You cut out desserts and begin a walking or gym routine. You feel much more energetic and alert because of your lifestyle change. But, when you step on your scale after the first month, you find that you have lost only six pounds, when you were expecting to have lost ten or more. In that one instant, all the self-esteem, enthusiasm, renewed clarity of mind, and joy you experienced from your daily walks deflate. You are left disappointed, maybe even hopeless. Your feeling of success evaporates, as if none of the benefits you enjoyed meant anything compared to an arbitrary figure on the scale.

This scenario is an example of the baffling ability we have to know and not know something at the same time. Surely, we can all see plainly how irrational it is to disregard our tangible experience of well-being in the face of not measuring up to a meaningless number! It's possible that this experience is the result of conflicting values. You have tagged the number on the scale with some emotional meaning so that you feel that nothing matters until you reach your goal weight, when everything in your life will fall into place. *That's* when you'll really be able to feel proud of yourself and to participate in the world like a "normal person."

What could inform a misguided belief like that? It may well be true that achieving a significant weight loss—or meeting any particular goal—will bring enormous benefits. However, it is important to delve into your belief that you don't deserve peace of mind until you achieve that goal. The practical, self-change reason for exploring this issue is that if your journey toward your goal is fraught with self-recrimination you are less likely to retain your focus and to make that journey (as I showed in Chapter 5).[1] Put simply, people don't like bad thoughts, even when they are used to motivate good behaviors. The further, PERFECT Program reason for reassessing your disappointment and gloom is simply that life comes with setbacks and disillusionments. But you are alive here and now, and the moment is precious.

What could be the underlying belief that causes you, or me, to tie our sense of accomplishment to an abstract number on the scale rather than to real, important benefits we have already experienced? It could be that—as I discussed in connection with self-acceptance—you feel you don't deserve to feel good about yourself unless you are a certain weight. The reason for your fixation with the scale number is that you aren't following your true values and priorities. There are two deductions from this example if it applies to you: first, to recognize that you are not measuring yourself by or following your own values and priorities; second, to explore whatever underlies your irrational perspective. This mindfulness exercise adds to the information you need to realign yourself with what's most important to you.

EXERCISE: When you consider your efforts to meet a goal or make a significant lifestyle change, can you remember a time when you were stymied or derailed by a setback? Why was that event so catastrophic? What were the underlying feelings that caused your extreme reaction? Do they seem reasonable in the light of day? What more genuine values of yours do they contradict?

Perfectionism

People—all of us—create perfectionistic goals that prevent us from really being who we can be and succeeding as best we can. Maybe it has even kept you from love, when you rejected a "non-perfect" relationship that was nonetheless loving and ultimately could have been highly fulfilling. At the same time, please keep in mind, reacting to an event like a possible "lost love" as a tragedy of unbearable enormity is a perfectionist response to the sin of perfectionism! If you have overcome the emotional pain and withdrawal of losing a love, don't add this additional, perpetual longing and grief reaction. (These reactions are not uncommon, it seems. I once was stuck at a workshop where each person was obligated to go up to everyone in the group and whisper what they wished they had told someone, but didn't. Every single person whispered in my ear: "I love you.") Now that it's done, carry on with your choice—there were, after all, reasons that caused you to choose as you did—and look for the love still available to you.

CASE: Willow ran an important nonprofit, inner-city agency. It had worthwhile goals, incredible challenges, and was underfunded and understaffed. Willow had never trained for a management position—she had started out as a volunteer. But soon her conscientiousness and commitment impressed everybody involved with the group—and she ended up heading the agency.

Willow was often depressed when she didn't accomplish all that she had hoped to. Nor were her tremendous efforts always appreciated in the welter of the city's and the agency's affairs. But everyone agreed that her impact was tremendously positive—that the agency had never functioned as well and done so much.

Nonetheless, Willow was seriously considering leaving her job—it was simply too draining. One day, as she left the public school where her office was housed, one of the kids who participated in Willow's program saw her leaving. He shyly came up to her, and said, "Miss ____. I have never been this happy in my life."

Willow realized instantly why she put up with the trials and tribulations of her work—that in many ways she was a rare and fortunate person.

Experiencing here-and-now rewards

As you go through your day, pursuing your goals, make it your plan to stop and recognize where you are and what you're doing that is different from what you would be doing were you still immersed in your addiction. For example, suppose you were accustomed to waking up with a painful hangover, piecing together details of the night before, but are now waking up refreshed. Take a moment before you get up to revel in the cozy feeling of being well rested and clear-minded in your bed, with nothing to regret. You may have farther to go. This period of sobriety may not turn out to be permanent. But allow yourself to realize that this is, indeed, a big deal, and how fantastic it feels. Meanwhile, don't lose sight of the "practical, self-change" reason for practicing these techniques while celebrating your good feelings in the moment. As we saw in Chapter 5, such self-rewarding makes it *much more likely* that you will progress, while self-criticism or lack of self-appreciation does the reverse.

If what you're doing during your day feels tedious—say you are filling out paperwork—acknowledge that you're doing something that is necessary, perhaps even important, in service of your larger goals. And when you're done, don't just move on to the next thing, as if nothing had happened. Reflect on this small triumph just to feel good about your day. If, beyond this, you meet a major milestone at work or in your personal life, celebrate fully. And especially do so when it comes to your addiction. Did you successfully navigate a trigger situation? Did you go a month without a drink? Did you finally do something that your addiction had always gotten in the way of?

Of course, although there are occasions when it's just the ticket, if you go out and buy yourself a present or treat yourself to a hot fudge sundae or a drink every time you accomplish something, this itself can be part and parcel of an addiction. But do allow yourself to revel in the satisfaction you derive from a job well done. Don't waste any opportunity to experience a sense of satisfaction. If you get on the scale and you've lost six pounds, if you can now walk around the block five times where previously you could only do it twice, if you aren't out of breath every time you climb the stairs the way you used to be—go with it! It's not everything you wanted—the whole enchilada—but it's a joy worth experiencing.

PERSONAL JOURNAL: When you go to bed, take a moment to list the pleasures, successes, and progress in your day. List at least five. Let the negatives take care of themselves.

EXERCISE: How many ways can you think of to acknowledge a success? For example, pausing to recognize it, calling a friend or supporter, or doing something special for yourself. Be as specific as possible, and try to practice these regularly. Make each a new habit, and even list these small celebrations on your tracking chart.

Honoring What You Value

Celebrating your successes is all about taking note of where you are at this moment and acknowledging how far you have come to get here. But there are valuable elements of your life that have remained constant, and recognizing those things on a daily basis (yes, you might call these "affirmations") is just as important. Giving yourself opportunities to remember who you truly are can help keep what's most important to you, and why you're doing what you're doing, in the forefront. This might include keeping photographs of people important to you where you can see them all the time—on your computer desktop, in your wallet, on your refrigerator. You might dust off the artifacts of your life that remind you of what's meaningful to you and place them prominently in your home—an instrument you used to (or still occasionally) love to play, a memento from a special trip or time in your life, a gift or card from someone you love.

ACTIVITY: Clear a space somewhere in your home—on a table or shelf or corner, perhaps close by your meditation spot. Gather some items that represent the best of who you are and what is most valuable to your heart. These could be childhood pictures of yourself or pictures of or items belonging to your children. You could include plants, candles, diplomas, creative works, products, religious symbols—as long as each represents an aspect of you and your life that brings you pleasure and a sense of value. Arrange these items in the space you have cleared, handling and placing your items with the intention of holding what each one symbolizes in your heart. Use this little altar as a touchstone—return to it whenever you can, to remember and meditate on what is truly meaningful to you.

But avoid fetishes

Your "values altar" is meant to be a guidepost for your life. As with the example of not making a fetish of the "lost love" that would have made your life okay, here, too, I should caution about the shrines some people keep with photos of dead parents, spouses, or children or long-lost lovers (sometimes under candlelight or small bulbs), or their school athletic trophies signifying things they can't do anymore and a kind of accomplishment and recognition they haven't since had. This kind of display can reinforce a negative focus on the past, against which the present and future look all the more bleak ("my best is behind me"). It is in the nature of balance that virtually every recommendation in *Recover!* carries with it a need to see the dangers in taking it to an extreme—in this case honoring things or people morbidly—and to be clear about the difference.

Going forward in honor

What is most important is that you honor your values, commitments, and love going forward. If there are people whose company you have neglected—perhaps feeling unworthy of their love—reach out. Schedule time with your family into your calendar, or commit to a weekly activity with your children. Contact an old friend. Seeing pictures of people important to you is nice, but actually contacting them from time to time is even better. You may have burned bridges in the past, or the people you love may be wary of opening themselves up to you again. In those instances it's important to respect their boundaries. Sometimes honoring someone you care about means giving them their space, while living in a way that reflects your feelings for them. Suppose, for instance, you have taken advantage of a good friend or a family member, and he cut you out of his life to protect himself from further harm. He or she plainly doesn't trust you, and there's nothing you can do about that (recall Harry and his daughter Anne in Chapter 5). Your decision to clean up your act does not obligate him to allow you back into his life, or even to hear your apology. You can still honor this person by changing your life and treating people the way you wish you had treated him.

Rituals, Traditions, and Celebrations

From the beginning of time, people have come together as families and communities to recognize and celebrate joyful or tragic events, rites of passage, milestones, harvests, the changing of seasons. Religious ceremonies, feasts, wakes, holidays, parties, rituals, and even more routine practices, like family meals, a kiss on the cheek before leaving the house, a weekly phone call, or a yearly block party are all part of the rhythm of life that makes us feel connected, part of something larger than ourselves. These events reinforce our human bonds, give structure to our lives, allow us to honor each other, our culture, and our humanity, and infuse our lives with meaning. This is yet another aspect of life that addicted people often neglect, opting out of gatherings where they won't have an opportunity to indulge or in order to isolate themselves, feeling ashamed to be around other people (remember Rose missing her daughter's party?), not feeling ties to their communities, or simply being unable to shift their focus away from the myopic and consuming involvement with addiction—and the empty rituals they share with fellow addicts.

Recognizing the profound importance of ritual can also be very personal and private, for instance, daily meditation or prayer or getting up early to watch the sun rise. Whereas previously your daily rhythm was driven by your addiction, you can now replace that frenetic, mindless activity with activities that draw you to life. Creating new personal rituals is a gentle place for you to start reconnecting. It allows you to enrich and fill your own life with a sense of reverence and respect for the world that surrounds you.

EXERCISE—CREATING RITUALS: Consider the ways you might begin introducing rituals into your personal or family life. Think about your daily schedule and what you can do to incorporate life-enhancing practices, like reading from an inspirational book or affirming your daily positives at bedtime; spending a few minutes mindfully exploring your values altar; or sharing an after-school snack with your child and talking about her day or reading to her in bed before she goes to sleep. Similarly, consider the more community-oriented rituals that you'd like to partake of, like joining a church or meditation group, attending community meetings, or walking with family or nearby friends after dinner. Begin making these occasions, these points of contact, a regular feature of your existence.

Traditions are family treasures. They are one of the touchstones that give us a sense of belonging and comfort. But, say, you are separated from your family or haven't inherited or don't practice any family or religious traditions. Then you can always start some yourself. For instance, some people volunteer at a soup kitchen on Thanksgiving or Christmas. Some families pass down a special heirloom on a significant birthday. A tradition can be as simple as a monthly Sunday dinner or as elaborate as a family reunion. Make a list of traditions, family or cultural, that are important to you, or traditions you would like to start. Perhaps you have seen others practicing a tradition that you found meaningful. Go on—steal it!

Commemorating major events with a celebration or remembrance is how we honor and attach value to one another—even when you throw a celebration for yourself. What better way to honor your friends and family than by asking them to share your significant life event? There are so many opportunities to celebrate: graduations, wedding or baby showers, birthdays, holidays, work promotions—significant recovery anniversaries. (AA has something there, although from the perspective of this book, as time goes on, that should fade in importance as you come to have more substantial, positive accomplishments and milestones.) Don't gloss over these events; instead, acknowledge them, whether by going out for dinner with a few special people, having a small party, or throwing a bash.

CASE: Richard had an ugly divorce, and his college-age son and adult daughter preferred being with their mother, who, after all, had always been the primary caretaker in the family. So Richard fiddled and fumed while he waited for his children to arrange get-togethers.

Once, as his birthday approached, it suddenly occurred to Richard that he could host his own party. He cleaned up his apartment, ordered some pizza and salad, and invited a couple of friends—along with his children and their dates. Although he was beset by anxiety about playing the unfamiliar role of host, the evening surprised Richard by being a resounding success.

As his son left, he told Richard, "That was great, Dad—let's do it again soon!"

Similarly, take the opportunity to grieve with others or share the sorrow of tragic events like deaths and illnesses. Sit Shiva or attend a wake; spend time with a friend with cancer. Being there for people is a major way of ensuring that you remain in the midst of humanity and acknowledge the humility of our existence in the universe. To put it in starker terms, we're all going to die. From The PERFECT Program perspective, appreciating the lives people have lived, their sheer presence on earth—which is the essence of mindfulness—gives your life a kind of immortality. In the words of John Donne: "Therefore never send to know for whom the bell tolls; it tolls for thee."

And while these ceremonies engage you with the people you cherish, they also impose on you accountability and responsibility to others, which is why it can be difficult for addicted people to participate in these activities. Anything that brings fulfillment to your life will push addiction away—and the flipside is also true: Neglecting these things will permit both the time and the psychic emptiness that invite vapid and destructive behavior. Rituals, traditions, and celebrations are not frivolous pursuits. They are essential, non-addictive links to your world.

Discovering Joy

Have you ever heard New Yorkers say they can always spot the tourists, because they walk around the city like rubes, with their mouths agape and their heads up, marveling at the sites and skyscrapers? For some reason, cynicism and world-weariness are considered admirable qualities in our culture, with "whatever" perhaps being the catchphrase of our era. Is reveling in a feeling of wonder a mark of lack of sophistication? I don't think so. (Although, as a New York resident, I *do* think Madame Tussauds is a rip-off and going up to the observation deck of the Empire State Building a waste of time for adults. Sorry.)

I'm going to speak now to your inner rube—the aspect of you that has been waiting around for an opportunity to be completely blown away by double rainbows and tall buildings. The pleasures and rewards of addictive behavior will blind you to joys you might never have known existed—or that couldn't hold your interest in the face of your addictive urges. How many opportunities to revel in something delightful have you missed? What beauty has escaped your notice? Now that you are headed down the path of your real life, you might feel as if you were blinking into the sun. Things you never noticed before might capture your attention and make you smile or marvel. I have written at length about linking yourself to the values that you know will bring joy and satisfaction to your life. Let's explore at the same time recognizing and discovering new joys. You cannot find too many ways of replacing the superficial rewards of addiction with the genuine rewards you gain from living a life of freedom.

CASE: When Thomas stopped smoking marijuana, he felt that he didn't know how to see and feel. After all, everything had been mediated by his being stoned—sometimes involving just staring at the wall! He found that there were two sides to this phenomenon. On the one hand, he had to immerse himself in appreciating every single aspect of every single day—including simply recognizing the passage of time, which being stoned hadn't permitted him to do. On the other hand, for the first time in a while he had the chance to indulge mindfully in the simple, pure joy of unadorned sensation and perception. In a way, "getting high on the natch" (natural) was the greatest trip of all.

Mindfulness in the wake of an addiction

We have discussed mindfulness as bringing unnoted reactions, emotions, and motivations to the surface of present consciousness. Thus, Thomas's story takes on a double meaning for mindfulness as a badge, a tool in recovery, particularly newly minted recovery.

CASE: At the time Liza quit drinking, after she had walked around in an alcohol haze for years, she really wondered what she was going to do with herself. Every single thing in her world had revolved around her drinking—every activity accompanied or was a precursor to drinking. In many cases, she had to learn for the first time the most basic aspects of having fun and filling her time—of living. After she had gotten beyond the miseries of quitting, she walked gingerly along the sidewalk, listening to the birds, watching the sun. It was a novel experience! She had to learn to be with people without alcohol, to go to the movies, to listen to music, and to do everything else stone cold sober. She began a list of things she could experience anew, some as simple as revisiting the supermarket. But there were also many new activities for Liza, like bike riding and cooking and sewing. She had plenty to choose from—it was as though she were a newborn.

Venturing away from addiction takes effort and focus—dealing with cravings, recovering after losing your footing, doing all these exercises, trying to be mindful. But even at the beginning of the journey, you may start noticing times when you're feeling pretty good or enjoying something you never bothered with before. For instance, on a walk, you might focus on the movement of your muscles working and enjoy the rhythm of your body, rather than thinking about the slog and how much longer it will take you to get home. (These are sensations encouraged by yoga and Feldenkrais, which I reviewed at the end of Chapter 4.) If you've stopped smoking, surely you'll appreciate the freshness of the air and your ease of breathing! Or, if you've given up drinking alcohol, you might notice how satisfying it is to down a cool glass of water. It could be that you never so much went to bed as passed out; now you are reminded of how good it felt to crawl under the covers as a child. There are an infinite number of ways to take pleasure in everyday life, and doing so is a choice and an exercise of mindfulness. In fact, if you pause right now, lift your head from your reading, you will surely be able to discover something that brings you some joy: perhaps you are feeling relaxed as you read or are sensing the sun on your skin, maybe there's a cat purring on your lap, or the tea you have next to you smells lovely. What do *you* notice?

Mindfulness en route to joy

Simply noticing and appreciating pleasant sensations or beautiful surroundings is one way of discovering joy. Another way is to intentionally seek out such sensations and surroundings. Make the effort to venture out into the world to create experiences that will bring you joy: Go for a hike through the park for no other purpose than to look around; smile at the people you pass; sit under a tree. Visit an unfamiliar part of town or go to another town or city; linger at shop windows; read the paper at a cafe. Or, staying closer to home, simply go out onto your step or into your back yard on a nice day to breathe deeply and smell the air and enjoy the sunlight on the trees. Staying indoors, read a book (okay, an e-book), or put on some new music. One way or another, open your heart and mind and senses to the world around you and acknowledge those things that inspire a sense of wonder or contentment. And before you fall asleep at night, recall those new experiences in as much detail as possible—especially the new joys they have brought you.

* * *

Much of your progress through The PERFECT Program has been on learning to cope with difficult feelings by strengthening your core, or inner wisdom and free will, and by replacing what is superficial and mindless with purpose, value, meaning, and mindfulness. It's a colossal effort, and the work you have been doing may bring you a real sense of satisfaction. One reason it may seem so hard to experience joy is our tendency to believe that we learn solely through difficulty and continuing trial. This tendency is strongly reinforced by the recovery movement mantra embodied by the white-knuckle phrase, "one day at a time." Just a reminder: Recovery—living—is more than not succumbing to addiction.

I believe—and I tell addicts—that they have been improved by the suffering and hardship they have endured—even if it was self-induced.

There are things you may know about yourself and life that you wish you hadn't had to learn, but that make you a deeper, more complete person now that you have. The lessons we learn from hardship are abiding and true. But they are far from the only truths you are going to gain in life. Understanding that some of your wisdom is hard won shouldn't make it harder for you to accept the wisdom that is earned through experiences of peace, satisfaction, fulfillment, and wonder. Shifting your perspective on this—toward valuing the insights you gain in joy as much as in hardship—is another way of bringing balance into your life. In short, knowing what works is even more important than knowing that addiction doesn't.

Putting It All Together

I've cited cases of mindful recovery earlier in this book. I want to end this phase of The PERFECT Program (before turning to the aftercare element presented by Chapter 10) with a case where a woman stabilized her life around a serious addiction—a set of addictions, really. This woman, Nona Jordan (whose program for women's financial self-management[2] is a resource referenced in Chapter 10), describes how she took control of her life over the long run, instituting changes that brought her a permanent set of rewards that finally guaranteed that her addictions would never reappear. Nona narrates her experience in her own words. The title of her case is her own.

CHANGE Is for Everyone Who Wants It

Lots of people are content with their lives and have no desire to change a thing. I've never been one of those people. My very earliest memories are of wanting to be my very best, to express the most perfect version of myself during this lifetime no matter what I'm doing.

In my late twenties, I was working in corporate accounting. I was good at the job but didn't really like it. I worked long hours and was constantly anxious about my performance. My favorite way of reducing stress was getting drunk at the local bar and smoking cigarettes until my throat hurt. Alcohol abuse is putting it mildly. Coming from a long line of alcoholics, I knew better—but it didn't stop me.

My relationships were disasters. The men I dated were poor choices and my friendships were all based on drinking. Despite my active social life, I felt isolated. I hid my drinking, which was getting harder to do. I was overweight from all the drinking. Drinking the way I was isn't cheap, either, and so I was in debt, even though I made a good living. I blamed others and my past for all of my problems.

It wasn't a pretty picture.

All this time, all through the drinking, I had continued to study and practice yoga and meditation. They seemed to be having very little benefit, but, little did I know, these practices were seeping into my life.

My moment of clarity arrived as the sun was setting one evening. I had finished a 6-pack already and was feeling ZERO effects from the beer. I was reading a book about Buddhism, which emphasized the idea of avoiding intoxication in order to clear away the cobwebs and experience life fully. As a way to really love yourself and grow from, and into, your life.

I looked up and I looked inward—I clearly saw the huge chasm.

Way over to the left was my current life: drunk, lonely, bad relationships, overweight, in debt, dissatisfied at work, no prospects in sight. Way over to the right was the life I knew I was meant to live: clear and happy, connecting to wonderful people in good relationships, healthy, helping others, doing work I love, with endless possibility for growth and change.

That night, I knew I was ready. I wanted to bridge that gap.

A few weeks later, I was sitting in the office of a Buddhist therapist that a girl at work had casually mentioned to me. It was my second day of not drinking and I felt horrible. But I knew if I was going to get the most out of therapy, I had to recognize my feelings. I was walking toward the version of me that I knew, deep down, I could be.

That was the beginning of the most life-altering, challenging, and—ultimately—profound period of my life. I broke up with my boyfriend. I stopped working so many hours (although, today, I work just as hard, only at gratifying things that I love). I started investigating yoga-teacher training programs. I started working out and honoring my body. I lost 30 pounds, almost effortlessly. I meditated; I got on my yoga mat and practiced for hours.

And I sat with my feelings and cried a lot. I worked hard with my therapist to clear away the rotten thoughts and beliefs that were mucking up my mind and my heart. I volunteered; I sought out healthy friendships; I paid off my debt.

I realized, in my heart—no, in my bones—that my life was my own. Happiness was in my hands, and my hands alone.

That was eleven years ago.

As of today, I am a married to a wonderful man and I have a beautiful daughter. I am a CPA, a yoga teacher, and a master coach. I work with women who want to create success on their terms. I have the pleasure of supporting them in finding the peace and ease that comes with creating a life and a financial legacy of their choosing.

My life is better than I would have ever imagined on that dark night so many years ago. There have been rough spots—really rough spots. This journey has not been easy, effortless, or flawless. But every year, I can say without fail, I more deeply love the life I have created for myself.

It's easy to say our situation is too hard, that someone else is holding us back, or that we're too damaged, broken, weak, or poor. But it's simply not true.

Life is what we make of it. Change is for anyone who wants it.

And that is the best news I can possibly give you on this fine day.

Moving Forward

You have learned the practice of The PERFECT Program for addiction, how to remove addiction from your life and replace it with genuine joy and accomplishment by homing in on your true self. You have learned to recognize and honor your success, to institute practices that reinforce and cement your ties to the things that make your life meaningful—your personal pleasures; your spiritual, familial, community, and cultural centers—and to cultivate new experiences of joy and wonder. Arriving at a place where you see the genuine value in celebrating your life in a way that is not narrowly self-involved and does not feel like a frivolous pursuit is a key stage in your recovery. This is this spirit that informs The PERFECT Program.

The following chapter is titled "Triage," which means dealing first with critical needs or circumstances, with emergencies. This is the chapter to turn to when you are feeling at a loss, or trying to remember your priorities in an overwhelming or difficult situation. It contains ideas and resources for dealing with cravings, relapse, life's curves, and other circumstances that require immediate guidance and perspective as you follow your new path.

CHAPTER 10

Triage

Realignment—Resources and actions for regaining lost footing

CHAPTER GOALS

- To deal with mishaps, discouragement, and persistent problems
- To plan for problem solving and realignment in the moment
- To review and consolidate the key ideas in The PERFECT Program
- To discover resources for support and exploration: helpful books, websites, meditations, and apps

Purpose: For moments when you feel overwhelmed or out of options, this chapter recaps key ideas, activities, and exercises from various parts of The PERFECT Program. It is a resource to give you quick reference points for shifting your perspective, moving forward, or regaining your footing. I also list other resources that can help you—some included in the previous chapters, some new—including books, websites, and guided meditations. If you find yourself at a loss, flip to this chapter, review your options, and pick a place to start. This is your on-the-spot reference and guide.

As you begin developing your skills and strengths, you may occasionally find yourself wondering how to get through the next moment without going off course. Perhaps you feel overwhelmed by urges, lost in the universe, unmotivated, depressed. This chapter is titled "Triage," which means dealing with the important things first, as they arise. This is a chapter that you can turn to when—whether having progressed this far in the program or not—you are feeling at a loss, or trying to determine what your priorities are in an overwhelming or difficult situation. These are ideas and resources for dealing with cravings, relapse, curves and dips in the road, and other events that require immediate guidance and perspective as you navigate the life of freedom you have created for yourself.

These ideas and resources can help you refocus in the moment. Some may not be for you; others might be just the thing. I will cover, in order:

- Difficulty with meditation
- Addictive urges and compulsions
- Relapse and harm reduction
- Feelings of unworthiness
- Lack of motivation
- Loneliness
- Feeling overwhelmed
- Anxiety or depression
- Abusive relationships
- Finding a therapist
- Education and career
- Financial management
- Other resources

Difficulty with Meditation

> *Mindfulness refers to keeping one's consciousness alive to the present reality. It is the miracle by which we master and restore ourselves.*
>
> —Thich Nhat Hahn

First, remember that meditation does not mean clearing your mind of all thoughts. Nor does it mean achieving total calm or enlightenment. Second, remember that the only right way to do it is to do it. Whatever *is* happening while you're doing your meditation is exactly what *should* be happening.

If you are experiencing pain, strong emotions, fidgeting, obsessing—meditation is not meant to alleviate those things. They are, in fact, your meditation companions—your guides, so to speak. To paraphrase Rumi, graciously invite in whatever devils show up—they all have something to teach you. So, before you begin, dispel any ideas you may have about what you should feel, how you should respond, what should happen. Whatever you feel, however you respond, and whatever happens is good.

Rather than teaching you to master your thoughts, feelings, or physical sensations, meditation is meant to help you master your ability to notice and accommodate them with compassion and a balanced perspective. Mindfulness is practice in paying attention to yourself, as well as in turning your attention where you will it. It is an exercise of your free will. It should be challenging, but when that challenge seems too much for you, here are some strategies you can implement. And, of course, I encourage you to search on your own for comparably valuable aids and resources.

- If you are having a hard time focusing your attention on your breath because you can't stop shifting and feeling antsy, turn your attention to those feelings instead of your breath. With a spirit of curiosity, explore that fidgety feeling: Where in your body is it located? Can you describe the sensation to yourself? Keep bringing your focus back to those feelings and notice what they do: Do they mutate? Do they intensify?
- Name what you're feeling, in your mind, as you experience it. Say to yourself, "Restlessness," "Thinking," "Ruminating," or "Listening to sirens outside." Once you have acknowledged what's happening, turn your attention back to your breath. Do this as many times as you need to. Your goal is not to prevent your mind from wandering. In fact, the heart of this practice is the intentional act of returning your attention to your breath as many times as required.
- Maybe, rather than feeling agitated, you experience a torpor that may mimic a deep, profound state of meditation. This can feel like a sinking into the mind, a dreamy heaviness that may even put you right to sleep! If you are experiencing this torpor and are unable to keep your mind alert, you can

meditate in an upright chair or do a walking meditation. You may also find it helpful to choose a basic guided mindfulness meditation CD or MP3.

- After the discussion here, review the section on mindfulness meditation in Chapter 4 ("Pause"), and particularly the section "User-Friendly Mindfulness Meditation" (page 98).

Resources for mindfulness meditation

BOOKS

Insight Meditation: A Step-by-Step Course on How to Meditate, by Sharon Salzberg

Mindfulness for Beginners: Reclaiming the Present Moment—And Your Life, by Jon Kabat-Zinn

The Miracle of Mindfulness: An Introduction to the Practice of Meditation, by Thich Nhat Hahn

AUDIO

How to Meditate: A Practical Guide to Making Friends with Your Mind, by Pema Chödrön

Mindful Movements, by Thich Nhat Hanh

Mindfulness for Beginners, by Jon Kabat-Zinn

WEBSITES

Audio Dharma: www.audiodharma.org (search for "Introduction to Mindfulness Meditation," by Gil Fronsdal)

U.C.L.A. Mindful Awareness Center: Free Guided Meditations http://marc.ucla.edu/body.cfm?id=22

University of Massachusetts Medical School Center for Mindfulness: Mindfulness Stress Reduction Programs: http://w3.umassmed.edu/MBSR/public/searchmember.aspx

Addictive Urges and Compulsions

If you do not change direction, you may end up where you are heading.

—Lao Tzu

If you are feeling overcome by strong addictive urges, you can shift your perspective in the moment by choosing one or a few of the following actions:

- **Mindfulness Meditation** with a focus on "Urge Surfing" (see "Guided Meditation," below).
- **S.P.O.T. Exercise,** Chapter 4 ("Pause," page 95).
- **Distract** yourself with an activity from the list you created in Chapter 7 ("Fortify," page 155).
- **Take a nap.**
- **Read an engrossing book.**
- **Eat a healthful snack,** like a handful of nuts or a piece of cheese or fruit.
- **Drink a full glass of water.**
- **Call a supportive, trusted friend.**
- **Walk.**
- **Bathe** and put on fresh, clean clothes.
- **Play some music** that is meaningful to you, either on a musical instrument or a recording.
- **Change your environment:** Go to a cafe, a friend's house, to the beach or park.
- **Start on a project,** something that has been waiting for your attention.
- **Give yourself permission** to use later (Chapter 7, page 158).
- **Remind yourself of your values:** Look at your photographs, explore your altar, pull out your lists of reasons to stay on track.
- **Watch a movie** that will make you laugh, or feel inspired by ideas and possibilities.

- **Consider the consequences:** Compose a story about what will happen if you indulge your addiction—from how it will make you feel in the moment all the way to the nearly inevitable consequences (depression, hangover, shame, etc.).

Resources for dealing with addictive urges and compulsions

BOOKS

Her Best-Kept Secret: Why Women Drink—And How They Can Regain Control, by Gabrielle Glaser

How to Change Your Drinking: A Harm Reduction Guide to Alcohol, 2nd ed., by Kenneth Anderson

The Mindfulness Workbook for Addiction: A Guide to Coping with Grief, Stress, and Anger that Triggers Addictive Behaviors, by Rebecca E. Williams and Julie S. Kraft

7 Tools to Beat Addiction, by Stanton Peele

Sex, Drugs, Gambling & Chocolate: A Workbook for Overcoming Addictions, by A. Thomas Horvath

The Tao of Sobriety: Helping You to Recover from Alcohol and Drug Addiction, by David Gregson and Jay S. Efran

The Truth About Addiction and Recovery, by Stanton Peele and Archie Brodsky

You Are Not Your Brain, by Jeffrey Schwartz

GUIDED MEDITATION

"Urge Surfing," by Sarah Bowen: http://depts.washington.edu/abrc/mbrp/recordings/Urge%20Surfing.mp3

COMMUNITY SUPPORT

HAMS, Harm Reduction for Alcohol: http://hamsnetwork.org

Moderation Management: http://www.moderation.org

SMART Recovery®: www.smartrecovery.org

Quit Smoking Support: http://www.quitsmokingsupport.com

We Quit Drinking: wqd.netwarriors.org

Relapse and Harm Reduction

> *When flowing water . . . meets with obstacles on its path, a blockage in its journey, it pauses. It increases in volume and strength, filling up in front of the obstacle and eventually spilling past it . . . . Do not turn and run, for there is nowhere worthwhile for you to go. Do not attempt to push ahead into the danger. . . (rather) emulate the example of the water: Pause and build up your strength until the obstacle no longer represents a blockage.*
>
> —Thomas Cleary, *I Ching*

You can be especially disheartened when you are in the thick of relapse, as the resolve you remember feeling seems so, so foreign and distant. But it is *always* within your power to regain your footing and focus. If you have relapsed, remember that there is no such thing as a "point of no return." Relapse is not evidence of failure or hopelessness. Your North Star is always in sight.

- Practice self-acceptance and compassion (see the following section on "Feelings of Unworthiness").
- Immediately begin employing harm-reduction techniques. Review in Chapter 3, pages 69–72.
- Review the section on relapse in Chapter 8, page 206.
- Remember that there is no such thing as starting over. If you have relapsed, broaden your perspective to see it as just a part of your whole journey to wellness.
- Remember that you can realign with your vision for yourself from any point, no matter how far off course you have traveled. Review the "Navigating Relapse" chart on pages 212–213.
- Take time to explore the circumstances or life events that may have triggered your relapse. Sometimes it's not clear, but more often you will be able to see exactly what triggered you to veer off course and why you were unable to steer through these

circumstances. Consider what you could have done differently and establish future coping strategies, in the highly likely event you encounter the same triggers again.

- Reintroduce The PERFECT Program into your daily life:
  - Begin practicing your mindfulness and loving kindness meditations, with an emphasis on riding out cravings and discomfort, in "Anti-Addiction Skills" section of Chapter 7, page 154.
  - Pay attention to your moments of grace and turn your attention to the messages you receive from your wise inner self.
  - Reconnect with your values and sense of life purpose and meaning in Chapter 6 ("Rediscover").
- Set some immediate goals.
  - Engage in the life-affirming activities you have created for yourself.
  - Consult "Reframing Failure," Chapter 8 ("Embark," page 204).
- Quick reference: Alan Marlatt's mindfulness-based relapse prevention S.O.B.E.R. exercise

S — *Stop:* pause wherever you are.
O — *Observe:* what is happening in your body and mind.
B — *Breathe:* bring focus to the breath as an "anchor" to help focus and stay present.
E — *Expand* awareness to your whole body and surroundings.
R — *Respond* mindfully versus automatically.

Dr. Marlatt explains:

S.O.B.E.R. is one of the meditation breathing spaces we've developed. You can use it when you're right on the verge of taking a drink. It enhances meta-cognition, giving you a chance to stand back and look at what's going on. Say you're walking by a bar you used to visit and the thought arises: "Maybe I'll just pop in and see if anybody I know is inside:" S is for "stop" where you are. Stop walking. Then O, "observe" how you're feeling—what are the physical sensations and cravings? B, focus on your "breath." Take a deep breath, then another breath, and center your attention there. And E "expand" your awareness so that you'll have a larger sense of what would happen if you did go in the bar. How would you feel? [. . .] Finally, R, "respond" mindfully.—Alan Marlatt, Interview, *Inquiring Mind*, 2010, www.inquiringmind.com /Articles/SurfingTheUrge.html.

Resources for understanding and dealing with relapse and harm reduction

BOOKS AND PAPERS

Addiction: A Disorder of Choice, by Gene Hayman

Enough! A Buddhist Approach to Finding Release from Addictive Patterns, by Chönyi Taylor

Harm Reduction Psychotherapy: A New Treatment for Drug and Alcohol Problems, by Andrew Tatarsky

How to Change Your Drinking: A Harm Reduction Guide to Alcohol, by Kenneth Anderson

Overcoming Your Alcohol or Drug Problem: Effective Recovery Strategies Workbook (Treatments That Work), by Dennis C. Daley and G. Alan Marlatt

Over the Influence: The Harm Reduction Guide for Managing Drugs and Alcohol, by Patt Denning, Jeannie Little, and Adina Glickman

Relapse Prevention: Maintenance Strategies in the Treatment of Addictive Disorders, by G. Alan Marlatt and Dennis Donovan

"Alcohol Harm Reduction Compared to Harm Reduction for Other Drugs," by Kenneth Anderson, http://hamsnetwork.org/9th-conference/compared.pdf

GUIDED MEDITATION

"Urge Surfing," by Sarah Bowen: http://depts.washington.edu/abrc/mbrp/recordings/Urge%20Surfing.mp3

WEBSITES

"The Clean Slate Addiction Site," by Steven Slate: www.thecleanslate.org

"HAMS: Harm Reduction for Alcohol": http://hamsnetwork.org

"Harm Reduction Network," by Kenneth Anderson: www.hamsnetwork.org

"How to Taper off Alcohol," HAMS Website: http://hamsnetwork.org/taper
"The Life Process Program," by Stanton Peele: peele.net
Moderation Management: http://www.moderation.org/
Quit Smoking Support: http://www.quitsmokingsupport.com
SMART Recovery®: www.smartrecovery.org
We Quit Drinking: wqd.netwarriors.org

Feelings of Unworthiness

> *You yourself, as much as anybody in the entire universe, deserve your love and affection.*
>
> —Buddha

I discussed at length in Chapter 5, on self-acceptance, knowing and believing that you are worthy of being in the world and of the things you value most, and that you have just as much right to create and participate in your own full life. Even the most seemingly well-adjusted people can feel unworthy to have these essential feelings. If you have trouble overcoming self-debasing thoughts or self-talk, or feel that you don't deserve love or success, please pursue some or all of the following suggestions:

- Reread the Chapter 5 section on self-acceptance (pages 116–120) and work through the exercises.
- Complete the self-compassion exercise, Chapter 5, page 118.
- Complete the self-forgiveness reflection, Chapter 5, page 122.
- Visit your altar or create one, Chapter 9 ("Celebrate," page 226).
- Reach out to someone who loves you.
- Practice your loving kindness meditation with dedication, Chapter 5, page 129, focusing specifically on self-compassion.
- Remember to write down five things you are grateful for, every morning or night.
- **Exercise:** In your Personal Journal, list the negative or harsh thoughts you are having about yourself or describe your negative feelings about yourself. Then review what you have written: Do you feel that you are fundamentally broken and irredeemable?

That you're a bad person? That you're not meeting expectations or goals? That you're less than everyone else? Now, explore your findings from a different perspective. Imagine that you are reading the words of someone you love—a child or close friend—or even a stranger. Does your self-assessment seem reasonable or realistic when you imagine directing these words at someone else? Rewrite your entry from this more compassionate perspective.

Resources for supporting feelings of self-worth

BOOKS

The Gifts of Imperfection, by Brené Brown
The Mindful Path to Self Compassion, by Christopher K. Germer
Radical Acceptance, by Tara Brach

GUIDED MEDITATIONS

"Lovingkindness Meditation," by Sharon Salzberg: www.soundstrue.com, www.sharonsalzberg.com
"Men, Women, and Worthiness," by Brené Brown: www.soundstrue.com, www.brenebrown.com
"Radical Acceptance Guided Meditations," by Tara Brach: www.tarabrach.com
All of the above meditations are also available from www.amazon.com.

WEBSITES

Befriending Ourselves, by Ali Miller: www.befriendingourselves.com
Self-Compassion, by Kristin Neff: www.self-compassion.org

Lack of Motivation

Nothing is a waste of time if you use the experience wisely.

—Auguste Rodin

A lack of motivation to act can seem like plain old laziness. But this paralyzing torpor is more likely generated by your fear, self-doubt, or irrational imagination. You may not know where to start, may be afraid of what you will discover if you start going through that pile of mail on your desk—or those feelings that await you just below the conscious level. Perhaps you can't bring yourself to start exercising, believing you'll just let yourself down in a couple of days anyway. You could be avoiding a phone call or work assignment, afraid of being judged or confronted in some way. Or you might just be exaggerating the potential tedium of whatever it is that you're avoiding. Granted, you may be right about all of it: Maybe there is a serious credit issue hiding in the pile on your desk; and maybe you do have an excruciatingly tedious task to face or an enormous project to tackle. Perhaps you're telling yourself that you're just waiting for the right moment or the right inspiration. Forget it. As Picasso said, "Inspiration exists, but it has to find you working." Let's get you moving:

- **Start small.** Give yourself only one task to accomplish for the day and commit to that single thing.
- **Give yourself a time limit**—say an hour or two—to work on a task. Buy and use a timer.
- **Use your tracking chart in your PERFECT Journal** to make note of everything you accomplished. Don't let this slide.
- **Choose an activity or event to attend** and put it on your schedule, even if it is for the following week. Make a coffee or walking date with a friend, find a volunteer opportunity, and so on.
- **Set a goal** and decide what steps you need to take to accomplish it. Break it down into mini-goals, then make a to-do list out of your mini-goals.
- **Write down the rewards** you will experience if you complete a task or project. For instance, how will you feel after making a dreaded phone call or cleaning your kitchen?
- **Find accountability in community.** Join a co-op or a book group; find an exercise partner or commit to helping someone.
- **Get showered and dressed for the day,** every day, even if you're not going somewhere.
- **Moments of grace.** Be mindful of and take advantage of your windows of opportunity to act. If you are surfing the Internet

and feel the sudden urge to shut it off and get up, do it. Don't wait for the feeling to pass.

- **Put on some motivating music or listen to a podcast or an audio book** when you're working on a boring chore that doesn't require your full attention.

Resources to help spark your motivation

BOOKS

Drive, by Daniel Pink
Getting Things Done, by David Allen
Making Habits, Breaking Habits, by Jeremy Dean
Willpower, by Roy F. Baumeister and John Tierney

AUDIO BOOKS/CDS

Getting Unstuck: Breaking Your Habitual Patterns and Encountering Naked Reality, by Pema Chödrön
The Willpower Instinct: How Self-Control Works, Why It Matters, and What You Can Do to Get More of It, by Kelly McGonigal: http://kellymcgonigal.com.

WEBSITES

"Flylady," www.flylady.net
"43 Folders," by Merlin Mann: www.43folders.com
"The Happiness Project," by Gretchen Rubin: www.happiness-project.com
"Procrastination," *Psychology Today*: http://www.psychologytoday.com/basics/procrastination
"Spark People," www.sparkpeople.com

OTHER

iTunes: Whether you have an Apple device or not, you can download iTunes, where you will find free music channels *and* podcasts on the subject of productivity. www.itunes.com

Loneliness

Be thine own palace, or the world's thy jail.

—John Donne

I've been lonely too long, I've been lonely too long / In the past it's come and gone. I feel like I can't go on without love.

—Eddie Brigati and Felix Cavaliere (The Rascals)

Loneliness is the devastating and painful emotional state of feeling alienated and isolated, which can be a powerful addiction trigger. You can experience loneliness whether you are physically alone or surrounded by friends, family, or community. After all, even connected people are often alone, or at least not immediately engaged with others (like working in an office cubicle). At the same time, you may not be in a committed relationship or part of any kind of larger community—at least in any immediate sense. Since our society is organized around couples and families, this kind of loneliness can make you feel as though you are especially deprived.

So, loneliness is a complex condition, with no single trigger—or even any trigger at all. People living with loneliness don't like to reveal it, because saying "I am lonely" is excruciatingly exposing and at the same time is easily dismissed as whining. But it's real, and it can be crippling.

Because loneliness is such a complex and persistent condition, patronizing instructions to get out and meet people don't help, especially because they don't take into account that many people who are plugged into communities can feel lonely. And, sometimes, forcing yourself into social situations can worsen feelings of isolation.

Most important to remember is that loneliness is not about other people; it's about your own sense of authenticity, your place and belonging in the universe. With that in mind, I offer these suggestions to help you restore or recognize your value and the vital nature of your existence.

- **Therapy:** Loneliness can lead to depression, addiction, even self-harm. If your loneliness is severe enough that you feel paralyzed or tempted to hurt yourself, please seek out effective treatment from a qualified therapist. See Chapter 7, page 163, Chapter 8, page 204, and "Finding a Therapist" later in this chapter for guidance in choosing a therapist.
- **Unplug:** Online networking has become a necessary part of daily life. We join online communities—like Facebook—or participate on message boards, where we communicate with people all day long. We text and instant message, e-mail, and remain accessible to everyone at all hours, and still the epidemic of loneliness grows. Remember that your body is more than just a vehicle to carry your brain around. Although sitting in front of your electronics all day can give you the illusion of connectedness or activity, you may be neglecting the plain fact that your body exists in this world, too. Connecting your body to the air, the ground, the weather, the food you eat—using all your senses every day—is essential to your feeling of belonging to this world. Consider scheduling time for your online social activities and making yourself less accessible. For instance, answer e-mail or text messages once or twice a day; turn on your instant messenger only for a limited amount of time; put your phone away when you are visiting with other people.
- **Volunteer:** Choose a cause that you believe in and offer your time and skills toward supporting it. Do so with the intention of engaging and furthering something meaningful to you. You might even find ways of spending time with other people who are lonely, like elderly neighbors or people who are housebound.
- **Reinforce your place in the universe:** Whether you are spiritually minded, agnostic, or atheist, you can find fulfillment in the rituals, practices, and philosophies that bring you a sense of your own meaning in the grand scheme. Find some meeting place for people with a spirit similar to yours—for meditation, yoga, hiking, church, or philosophical discussions.

- **Find a regular place for yourself:** Go somewhere regularly, to work or to socialize or to sit and think. This can be a park, or a coffee house, or—yes—even a nice bar. Although this contradicts the idea of feeling lonely by being alone in a crowd, there is a point to "having a place."
- **Share your knowledge:** What skills do you have that you can share with others? Can you teach someone to sew? Garden? Do algebra? Fish? Offer to teach someone how to do something that you are good at, even if you are not an expert!
- **Practice your loving kindness and compassion meditations and skills** from Chapter 5, with the intention of extending these feelings outward, to your friends, family, community, and further toward acquaintances, people you see daily, and even people you don't like.

Resources to help you cope with loneliness

Review the resources for "Feelings of Unworthiness," page 247.

BOOKS

Living Single, blogs and books by Bella DePaulo: http://www.psychologytoday.com/experts/bella-depaulo-phd

Lonely: Learning to Live with Solitude, by Emily White

True Belonging: Mindful Practices to Help You Overcome Loneliness, Connect with Others, and Cultivate Happiness, by Jeffery Brantley and Wendy Millstine

Feeling Overwhelmed

> *You are the sky. Everything else—it's just the weather.*
>
> —Pema Chödrön

Feeling overwhelmed is the sense that you are out of control, either of a situation or of your emotional response to it. It's the feeling that you are in way over your head, or that you cannot think rationally or act effectively. Perhaps you don't know where to begin tackling a big problem and have been allowing it to spiral into chaos. Or, perhaps you have too much on your plate. It could also be that you are so overcome by emotions that at this moment you cannot act effectively or think rationally. Anger, fear, stress, grief, exhaustion, and trauma can all contribute to the belief that you have no options. Here are some places to start:

- **Mindfulness meditation:** This is essential for gaining and maintaining rational perspective, for centering yourself and finding repose.
- **Delegate:** Ask for help.
- **Break it down:** Dismantle any huge tasks into more manageable mini-tasks, and pick a place to start.
- **Take a break:** Remove yourself from any volatile or emotionally fraught situation until you regain some control or perspective.
- **Listen:** Talk through the situation with a friend or therapist. Remember to really listen to feedback and keep your mind open to possibilities. Resist the urge to say "Yeah, but . . . " and to dismiss options that have been presented to you. You don't have to follow through on everything you hear, but keep an open mind and make sure you are listening.
- **Create opportunities:** Make a list of potential options and decisions you can make about your situation, especially if you're feeling stuck. Do this with a friend or helper, if possible.
- **Review problem-solving skill:** Chapter 7 ("Fortify," page 166).

Resources for helping you regain control when you're feeling overwhelmed

BOOKS

Calming the Emotional Storm, by Sheri Van Dijk
Emotional Intelligence 2.0, by Travis Bradberry and Jean Greaves
True Refuge, by Tara Brach
When Things Fall Apart, by Pema Chödrön

AUDIO

Don't Bite the Hook: Finding Freedom from Anger, Resentment, and Other Destructive Emotions, by Pema Chödrön
Living Without Stress or Fear, by Thich Nhat Hahn
Stress-Proof Your Brain, by Rick Hanson

WEBSITES

"Wisdom through Mindfulness": wisdomthroughmindfulness.blogspot.com

Anxiety or Depression

> *This being human is a guest house. Every morning is a new arrival. A joy, a depression, a meanness, some momentary awareness comes as an unexpected visitor . . . . Welcome and entertain them all. Treat each guest honorably. The dark thought, the shame, the malice, meet them at the door laughing, and invite them in. Be grateful for whoever comes, because each has been sent as a guide from beyond.*
>
> —Rumi

Anxiety and depression are common mental health issues; they can cast a shadow over your life and make it difficult to maintain perspective or focus on your daily activities. As your mind and body adjust to your non-addicted way of life, you may experience periods of depression or anxiety. Avoiding these feelings can make reverting to addiction seem like the lesser of two evils. Remember that these feelings will likely pass—or come and go—but to make life bearable while you are in the thick of it, you can take steps to see you through them.

- **Therapy:** If your anxiety or depression is chronic and severe enough to be debilitating, please visit a therapist who specializes in depression and anxiety. See "Finding a Therapist" later in this chapter for guidance on choosing a therapist.
- **Go outside:** Expose yourself to the elements for at least fifteen minutes a day.
- **Clean and declutter** your immediate environment.
- **Stay on your schedule.**
- **Reframe:** In your journal, write down the thoughts you are having about yourself or your situation and ask yourself how

realistic or accurate those thoughts are. Have a friend help you, if possible.

- **Eat healthfully:** Get rid of the junk food and sugar. If you're anxious, cut out caffeine.
- **Change your environment:** Go somewhere open and peaceful, if that is a possibility for you. Head to a park or to a lake or ocean beach and absorb the new scenery. Or go downtown and people watch or window shop.
- **Move:** Dance, exercise, walk the dog, ride your bike, swim, stretch. It doesn't matter what you do, but do something with your body.
- **Consume information wisely:** Choose the media you consume with intention. Turn off the violence, the exploitative reality TV shows, and gossip. Avoid vitriolic Internet comments sections and mindless, time-sucking websites. Limit your media exposure, focusing your attention on what is informative, uplifting, inspirational, thought-provoking, and creative. Get your current events news from reliable sources such as a daily newspaper and/or public radio.

Resources for managing depression and anxiety

THERAPY

Review "Find Professional Help": Chapter 7, page 163
Review "Mental Health" (including types of therapy): Chapter 8, page 204
See "Finding a Therapist" later in this chapter.
Hakomi (meditation-based) Psychotherapy: http://hakomiinstitute.com/about/the-hakomi-method

BOOKS

Feeling Good, by David D. Burns
The Mindful Way Through Depression, by Mark Williams and John Teasdale
The Mindfulness Solution: Everyday Solutions for Everyday Problems, by Ronald Siegel
Psychotherapy Without the Self: A Buddhist Perspective, by Mark Esptein
When Panic Attacks, by David D. Burns

GUIDED MEDITATIONS

Free Yourself from Anxiety, by Erin Olivo: soundstrue.com

"Guided Forgiveness Meditation for Depression," by Ronna Kabatznick, free from Audio Dharma: www.audiodharma.org

"Relieve Depression," by Belleruth Naparstek: healthjourneys.com

AUDIO

The Fearless Heart: The Practice of Living with Courage and Compassion, by Pema Chödrön

Living Without Stress or Fear, by Thich Nhat Hahn

MIND-BODY ACTIVITY WEBSITES

Gaiam: www.gaiam.com

Feldenkrais Method: www.feldenkrais.com

MINDFULNESS PSYCHOTHERAPY WEBSITES

The Institute for Mindfulness and Psychotherapy: http://www.meditationandpsychotherapy.org

The Mindfulness Solution:
http://www.mindfulness-solution.com

Mark Epstein on Mindfulness and Psychotherapy
http://www.psychotherapy.net/interview/epstein-buddhism

Abusive Relationships

> *Never allow someone to be your priority while allowing yourself to be their option.*
>
> —Mark Twain

Living with abuse, mental or physical, including infidelity, is traumatizing and crazy-making. If you are being manipulated, bullied, lied to, intimidated, emotionally or physically abused, you can lose your faith in yourself, your sense of self-worth, and your ability to recognize and act on the real options you have—all of which can reduce your ability to cope with addiction. If you are suffering with abuse, in any form, *it is vital* that you remove yourself from the harmful, traumatizing domestic or social situation.

Escaping abuse is much easier said than done when your finances or livelihood or sense of self-worth are dependent on your abuser, or when you have been so devastated that you don't trust yourself to make the proper choices. It may seem a paradox to say that your sense of self-worth is (or feels as though it is) dependent on the abuser. Yet, this is the basic dynamic in an addictive, abusive relationship—abuse and dependence feed on one another. Clearly, the subjects of addictive and abusive relationships can be the basis for an entire book (like *Love and Addiction*). For the present purpose of avoiding falling back into an addiction, let me offer here some guidance and resources that can help you find support and sanctuary.

- **Reach out to family and friends:** Often, people who are being abused are ashamed to admit it to the people closest to them, for a variety of reasons. Abusers also will take measures to isolate their victims from family and friends. It is important that you let your loved ones know what is happening to you. Not only will this allow people to help you, it will also bring you a sense of accountability to people outside of your abusive circumstances.
- **Contact domestic abuse support:** Local shelters, abuse hotlines, police, and courts can advise you and provide you with a supportive network.
- **Remember who you are:** People who are being abused often lose their sense of self, forgetting what inspires them and brings their life meaning. Removing yourself from an abusive environment, changing your physical perspective, even for a short time, can help ground you and remind you that the world is bigger than your immediate situation.
- **Value, purpose, and meaning:** Review Chapter 6 ("Rediscover") to reestablish your priorities.
- **Counseling:** Find a counselor or therapist who specializes in abuse. Be alert for and wary of people who use buzzwords and phrases like "codependency" and "look at your part." For sure, you want to explore the reasons why you might find yourself accommodating an unacceptable situation, but do so with someone who is not locked into a 12-step philosophy. (See the next section of this chapter, "Finding a Therapist.")

- **Review my discussion of permission in "Self-Knowledge and Personal Choice" (Chapter 8, page 188):** Remember that abusers (like addicts) don't abuse (or make poor choices) because they're "passionate" or "out of control." We all go only as far as we have given ourselves permission to go.
- **Review "Boundary Setting" (Chapter 7, page 176):** In essence, abuse is the failure to observe boundaries. Your boundaries—or where you end and others begin, what you will or will not permit others to do to you (or what you will do to them)—are critical in abuse.

Resources for dealing with abusive situations

BOOKS

Although many books on abuse speak directly to women—since 85 percent of abuse victims are women—these should not be dismissed by men who are living with abuse:

Love and Addiction, by Stanton Peele with Archie Brodsky
The Verbally Abusive Relationship: How to Recover, by Patricia Evans
Why Does He Do That? Inside the Mind of Angry and Controlling Men, by Lundy Bancroft

GUIDED MEDITATIONS

"Guided Meditations for Self Healing," by Jack Kornfield: www.jackkornfield.com, www.soundstrue.com
"Heartbreak, Abandonment, and Betrayal," by Belleruth Naparstek: www.lifejourneys.com
"Meditations for Emotional Healing," by Tara Brach: www.soundstrue.com, www.tarabrach.com
The meditations above are also available at www.amazon.com and itunes.

WEBSITES

National Domestic Abuse Hotline: www.thehotline.org. This website contains a wealth of information, resources, links, support, and guidance.

Finding a Therapist

If you believe it would be helpful to seek therapy for support in overcoming addiction or other mental health or emotional issues, here are some tips on finding someone who suits you. You are seeking someone who is qualified to address your particular problem areas, who is not locked into an agenda at odds with your own, whose point of view is simpatico with your values, and whose opinion you respect.

- **Get referrals:** Ask trusted friends who share your sensibilities and worldview for recommendations.
- **Research:** Go online and read client reviews or visit therapists' websites and read their philosophies and writing.
- **Interview:** Your relationship with your therapist is an important one. Remember that you are seeking to hire someone for a service, and not everyone will possess the specific skills or perspective you are looking for. Inquire whether they offer free initial consultations, or at least speak with them by phone. Before you go in or speak with the person, make note of what qualities are important to you in a therapist. Ask questions about his or her approach and philosophy. Keep interviewing until you find someone who is a good fit for you.
- **Ask about payment:** Some therapists will take insurance, others will offer a sliding scale to low-income clients. Ask about your options.
- **Trust your gut:** Therapists will often encourage their clients to venture out of their comfort zone, which is appropriate. However, it's important for you to distinguish between challenging yourself and violating your values. It is a red flag if a therapist instructs you to do something that offends or compromises your values. Immediately express your reservations. Don't be pressured into doing anything you don't believe is right. If you are feeling bullied or manipulated, the odds are that your feelings are correct. Trust yourself and move on.
- Review "Boundaries and Addiction Treatment" in Chapter 7 (page 180), "Find Professional Help" in Chapter 7 (page 163), and "Mental Health," including types of therapy, in Chapter 8 (page 203).

Resources to help you find a therapist

Hakomi (meditation-based) Psychotherapy: http://hakomiinstitute.com/about/the-hakomi-method

Inside Rehab: The Surprising Truth About Addiction Treatment? and *How to Get Help That Works,* by Anne M. Fletcher

Psych Central, Therapist Directory: http://psychcentral.com/find-help

Psychology Today, Therapy Directory: therapists.psychologytoday.com

Education and Career

The PERFECT Program is based on the belief that you will overcome addiction when you connect with your true self instead of an addiction, follow your values and the purposes these lead to, and pursue the resulting goals you select. Any other form of addiction therapy or resolution is stopgap, and cannot have the fundamental link to your heart and mind that true recovery requires. Following are resources for pursuing your education and desired job or career.

If you are considering going back to school, but don't know where to start, let me offer you some practical help:

- If you need to earn your GED (General Education Diploma), visit the GED Testing Service website (www.gedtestingservice.com) to find resources and information. You may even contact them by phone or e-mail to get help.
- Stay away from the for-profit colleges you see advertised on TV. They're extremely expensive, their standards are low, and they are not as successful at finding placement for their graduates as established educational institutions.
- Ask yourself if you want to pursue a degree or a trade.
- Choose a few areas that interest you and that you believe you have an affinity for, and that might be a practical choice for your future. For instance, you might love philosophy, but consider what positions that field of study will qualify you to hold once you have earned your degree.
- Get online and see if there are any local schools that offer what you are looking for.

- Contact the schools and make an appointment with their admissions adviser or the adviser for the particular program or degree you are interested in.
- Before your meeting, make sure you have a list of questions and goals, so that they can guide you effectively toward meeting or reassessing your goals.
- There are many options for funding. Make an appointment with the Financial Aid office. You might find that you qualify for a loan, scholarship, or grant.
- If you are short on time, check to see if your school offers online courses or night courses, as well as child care.

If your goals are occupation-oriented—say you would like to work in a particular field, seek promotion in your current job, or even start your own business—there is guidance and resources for you, too.

- Many community colleges offer career-counseling services for students.
- Visit your state's government page (which will normally be www.[fillinyourstate].gov and seek out their Employment Services under their Human Services Department. You might discover that your state has what's called "Vocational Rehabilitation," which provides counseling in all aspects of finding employment.
- A well-composed resume is required. Find a professional resume-writing service that can provide you with a neat, thorough resume. It is worth the money.

If you are seeking to advance in your current employment, there are several approaches you can take:

- Complete your Goals Worksheet, but include some time-specific goals: for instance, where would you like to be in a year's time, five years' time? What will you have to do to meet these goals (e.g., more education or training)? Find out if your company will cover all or some of the costs of your further education.
- Make contact with others at your employment who have already met the goals that you have set for yourself, and ask them for guidance.

- Do the best job you can do in your current position.
- Keep your ear to the ground and ask around, at work and on the outside! You might find that another business can offer you more opportunities for advancement.

Perhaps you are interested in starting your own business. How do you go about that?

- The first thing to do is to contact your local Small Business Association. They offer free business counseling, no matter what stage you are in—even if you are just contemplating the idea. They also offer classes in several areas, from bookkeeping to preparing an effective business plan.
- Speaking of business plans: This is a crucial step, even if you have no intention of presenting it to a bank for a loan. Doing so will help you clarify your goals and recognize whether or not you are being realistic.
- Start small and let your business grow organically. There is always the temptation to throw all your time and money into a new business, because it's so exciting. However, there is a lot to learn along the way, and you don't want to miss those lessons—or find yourself in too far over your head and in debt before you have an opportunity to make effective adjustments.
- Do your research. This does not mean simply buying a book. Talk to others who are running businesses like the one you want to create. (You know the definition of an expert? Someone who has already done what you want to do.) If you have the opportunity, work for one of these businesses, so you can experience their reality.
- Based on your goals, values, and journal exercises, examine whether it is realistic for you to devote yourself to the type of business you have in mind.

Financial Management

Finally, no other strictly practical matter will sidetrack you from achieving recovery the way financial distress can do. Likewise, financial distractions will undermine your life goals almost as much as will legal, health, family, and emotional problems. Yet—of these things—finances are the easiest to control through limited, but concentrated, effort. So let's tackle finances and restore your peace of mind. No matter how much of a mess you have on your hands, you can pull yourself out of it and keep yourself out. Schedule time on your calendar to devote to this. When that time comes, shut off your phone, iPad, and so on, and then break this task down into a series of manageable mini-goals.

- Organize all your bills. This process of organization should help you gain some clarity and sense of control over your situation. Even if you find that you are more in debt than you expected, or are overwhelmed by what you must face up to, you have taken an enormous step forward, and there is support available to help you prioritize and tackle your financial issues.
- If you have unopened mail and bills accumulating around your house or on your desk, put them all in one place. Find a container—perhaps a paper bag or a box—to put everything in.
- Once you have everything in one place, you're going to sort through it. Clear a workspace for yourself, perhaps a kitchen table or even the floor, and create two categories: Save and Discard. In your Save pile, put all the bills or paperwork that you will need to deal with either right away or at some point in the future, and then items you should file away. In the Discard pile, include everything that is redundant (save only the most recent of each type of bill). Be careful about how you dispose of the material in your Discard pile, because it may contain sensitive information. If you have access to a shredder, use it. Remove the Discard pile from your workspace as quickly as possible, to get it off your mind.
- Now, you will want to break down your Save pile into a few more categories. Again, clear your workspace of clutter, especially your Discard pile. Your categories here will include items you can deal with immediately—for instance, bills you can afford to pay on the spot; items you must take further action on or get more information about before they can be dealt with—for instance, you may have to make a phone call about payment arrangements; and items that must be filed. So: Now; Later; and File.

- In a notebook, create a checklist that corresponds to each pile. For the Now pile, simply create an entry for each item. For the Later pile, create an entry for each item, and underneath it write down the steps you need to take. If you have phone calls to make, copy down the contact information, your account number, how and when you will contact the debt-holder or other party, how much you owe, or any relevant information you'll need to take those further steps. You may be aware of financial obligations for which you have no paperwork on hand. Add these to your list, along with the steps you need to take to find out exactly what to do. For your File pile, examine your items one by one and determine what categories they belong in: financial statements, receipts, credit card statements, mortgage statements.
- If there is anything you can handle right now, do it, and check it off your list.
- Speak to a debt counselor. Now that you have a better handle on your situation and understand what needs to be addressed, you will have the information you need to present to a counselor who can help you. Be wary of the "debt consolidation" services you hear advertised on TV or radio. Instead, seek out an accredited, nonprofit organization whose counselors can mentor you in budgeting without ulterior motives. Check out the National Foundation for Credit Counseling (www.nfcc.org) to find counseling in your area. They offer a wealth of information and guidance in several areas of financial concern.
- If you would like to know what your credit score is, be similarly wary of the businesses you see advertised. They may say they offer free information, but you often can find yourself paying for unnecessary information or services. All three credit-reporting agencies are required, by law, to provide you with a free copy of your credit report and score once a year, and they have set up a website where you can request your reports—www.annualcreditreport.com. The best place for you to start is at the Federal Trade Commission website—www.ftc.gov—where you will find the clearest instructions.
- Avoid predatory lenders! That includes car title loan businesses, check-cashing services, and car dealers or other businesses that

promise to finance anyone, "Bad Debt OK!" These businesses exist solely for the purpose of putting you further into debt and ruining your credit. That, in fact, is their business plan. They exist to prey on desperation. There are always other options, including the following.

- Contact your creditors for a payment arrangement. Utility companies, for example, normally will do everything they can to prevent cutting you off, if you are simply willing to make the phone call. Credit card companies likewise are motivated to arrange a "workout." Don't ask how I know such things, which are explained at http://banking.about.com/od/loans/p/workout.htm.
- Contact your local social services organization. It's possible they can provide you with emergency help.
- Make an appointment with the Credit Counseling Service, who may be able to direct you to other resources.
- Seek the services of a reputable financial adviser or a group that works with people like you, and that is not oriented primarily towards hijacking additional fees from you. Such resources exist, as represented by Nona Jordan in the previous chapter: nonajordan.com.
- Do not be afraid or ashamed to ask for help from friends or family or your church, if this is an option for you. They may be glad to help you in the service of your larger goals.
- Implement a system: Create an inbox dedicated only to your bills, and carve out a time every month for taking action on each item. Have envelopes, stamps, pens, a calculator, and whatever other items you may need to facilitate the task. You can set up automatic bill-paying through your bank for almost any service you pay for, from your utilities to your credit card bills.
- Review your bank statement regularly to determine whether there are any recurring expenses that you can't afford. For instance, perhaps in a state of inebriation you signed up for an online service and then promptly forgot about it! Are you being charged monthly for anything you're not using? (Again, something we all might know about.) Perhaps your bank is debiting a monthly service charge from your account that you were unaware of.

- If you are technically adept, you can consider exploring a free money-management system, like mint.com, which allows you to set spending limits, make up a household budget, send yourself alerts when bills are coming due, and receive notifications when your balance is getting low or when you have been charged a service fee.
- Explore free classes in money management.
- Find books online, at the library, or at your local bookstore about basic financial management.
- Really, it will all work out—they no longer have debtors' prisons. Note: For relief take Dickens's *Little Dorrit*—DVD or book—out from your local library, or read online (http://charlesdickenspage.com/dorrit.html). Don't buy a copy of this or any other book or DVD (except for *Recover!*) and any other practical guides or make any other nonessential purchases.

Beyond This Chapter—And the Book

This chapter gives you a quick, comprehensive overview and ideas for managing various life circumstances that you may have difficulty coping with during your recovery. It is also worthwhile to create your own personal "Triage" list, based on your experience, focusing on areas you expect you will have trouble with and solutions you believe will work best for you. If you find that a challenge you anticipate was not covered in this chapter, you might still peruse the lists and resources I have provided. But if you cannot find what you're looking for, I encourage you to explore on your own. Get online. Local and state government agencies offer you public resources. Don't be afraid to make phone calls and ask questions, request direction, or ask for referrals. Pursuing resources on your own is an empowering exercise of the life skills—of the life outlook—that The PERFECT Program is about.

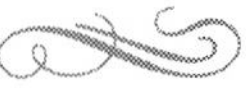

Afterword

Write Your Own Conclusion

Recover! is a title in the form of an imperative—something that you *should* do. But this book tells you not to follow other people's scripts or philosophies other than those you develop for yourself from your own experience. You can abstain or moderate or curtail harms; you can join groups—religious, AA, or otherwise—or go it on your own. You can meditate while sitting upright, standing, walking, or—from a yoga position—standing on your head.

In telling you that how you proceed from here is up to you, I am simply stating the obvious. Still, I want you to get better—to improve your state of mind, your life, your relationship to the people and the world around you, and to cease your addiction(s). But I want to send you off with more than good wishes. I want to remind you of all that you have accomplished by thinking about addiction and learning and practicing The PERFECT Program.

You began with deep concerns about yourself and your life. And you have embarked on a journey to recover your real self, the person you are capable of being, based on your values and purpose. This is the meaning of your existence—much of which is already in place, perhaps for you to be reminded of, some of which it is yet for you to discover. As well as rediscovering who you are, you have developed the tools and skills to lead a positive, non-addicted lifestyle. You have worked on focusing your mind in new ways while accepting your true self as part of your permanent, true recovery; you have practiced communication, listening, and problem-solving skills, including how to quit your addiction and maintain your freedom; you have developed plans both for daily living and for your future—including how you deal with work, finances, intimacy, your family; how you will spend your "free" time and with whom; and what your life goals are and will be. That's effort well spent.

You have learned through The PERFECT Program to be mindful of yourself and your world, to embrace your inner being and real self, to breathe easily, not to panic, to keep your goals and techniques in mind, and to move carefully but resolutely ahead. You have also learned two essential things. The first is to celebrate your existence on earth, to take full advantage of and appreciate this world and all that it contains—people, nature, opportunities, pleasure, yourself.

Which leads to the second key thing that you have learned. You can—you must—count on yourself—look to yourself as your own best advocate, supporter, and friend. You have been engaged in imagining and planning your life after reading this book. Now you must navigate that life. This isn't a command I'm giving you—it's a statement of an inevitable reality. No one else can pilot your life for you—at least if you are following The PERFECT Program.

There are many other people in your life who are wishing you well besides me and Ilse Thompson. For one thing, you can seek support and have contact with fellow travelers on this voyage—and this does *not* mean simply those who have suffered addictions identical to your own. There are *many* people for whom you are becoming a new, non-addicted person—children, spouses, partners, parents, teachers, faith leaders, friends, extended family, members of communities you choose to become part of—all of whom will benefit from, and deeply appreciate, who you are becoming.

I wish you a good journey as you go forth to realize your potential. This is not always a safe and sure journey—there are rocks and turns on every path. But it is a journey that you are capable of making and that you will make—sooner or later. The PERFECT Program is just a road map to make that passage a little quicker and easier.

Now carry on with my and Ilse's best wishes,

Stanton Peele and Ilse Thompson
Co-Founders, The PERFECT Program

Notes

Introduction

1. Centers for Disease Control and Prevention, *Smoking Cessation*. National Center for Chronic Disease Prevention and Health Promotion: Office on Smoking and Health, 2012, http://www.cdc.gov/tobacco/data_statistics/fact_sheets/cessation/quitting/index.htm.

Chapter 1

1. Carl Hart's book, *High Price: A Neuroscientist's Journey of Self-Discovery That Challenges Everything You Know About Drugs and Society* (HarperCollins, 2013), details the myths surrounding drugs, and particularly meth, whose uncontrollable, brain-destroying effects Hart's research contests. Hart "even takes on 'meth mouth,' noting that the dry mouth symptoms that have been blamed for the terrible dental problems seen in some methamphetamine users also accompany the use of legal amphetamines and some antidepressant medications." Maia Szalavitz, "Why the Myth of the Meth-Damaged Brain May Hinder Recovery," *Time Healthland*, November 21, 2011, http://healthland.time.com/2011/11/21/why-the-myth-of-the-meth-damaged-brain-may-hinder-recovery.

Chapter 2

1. Hillel R. Alpert, Gregory N. Connolly, and Lois Biener, "A Prospective Cohort Study Challenging the Effectiveness of Population-Based Medical Intervention for Smoking Cessation," *Tobacco Control*, January 10, 2012, http://tobaccocontrol.bmj.com/content/early/2012/01/03/tobaccocontrol-2011–050129.abstract.

2. Jacqueline Detwiler, "The Ten Hardest Drugs to Quit," *The Fix*, December 20, 2011, http://www.thefix.com/content/10-hardest-addictive-drugs-to-kick7055.

3. Stanton Peele, "Proof That Treating Addiction with Drugs Doesn't Work," *Huffington Post*, January 11, 2012, http://www.huffingtonpost.com/stanton-peele/smoking-addiction_b_1195953.html.

4. Benedict Carey, "Nicotine Gum and Skin Patch Face New Doubt," *New York Times*, January 9, 2012, http://www.nytimes.com/2012/01/10/health/study-finds-nicotine-gum-and-patches-dont-help-smokers-quit.html.

5. Lindsey F. Stead, Rafael Perera, Chris Bullen et al. "Nicotine Replacement Therapy for Smoking Cessation," *The Cochrane Library,* November 14, 2012, http://onlinelibrary.wiley.com/doi/10.1002/14651858.CD000146.pub4/abstract.

6. Brad W. Lundahl, Chelsea Kunz, Cynthia Brownell et al., "A Meta-Analysis of Motivational Interviewing: Twenty-Five Years of Empirical Studies," *Research on Social Work Practice* 20(2):137–160, 2010.

7. Stanton Peele, *The Meaning of Addiction*, 2nd ed. (San Francisco: Jossey-Bass, 1998); http://lifeprocessprogram.com/the-meaning-of-addiction-1-the-concept-of-addiction.

8. American Psychiatric Association, *APA Corrects New York Times Article on Changes to DSM-5's Substance Use Disorders* (Arlington, VA: American Psychiatric Association, 2012).

9. Stanton Peele, "Addiction in Society: Blinded by Biochemistry," *Psychology Today*, September 1, 2010, http://www.psychologytoday.com/articles/201010/addiction-in-society-blinded-biochemistry.

10. See "The Amen Solution," http://www.amenclinics com/?p=5158&option=com_wordpress&Itemid=204.

11. Mika Brzezinski, *Obsessed: America's Food Addiction—And My Own* (Philadelphia: Weinstein/Perseus, 2013).

12. Michael Moss, *Salt Sugar Fat: How the Food Giants Hooked Us* (New York: Random House, 2013).

13. Stanton Peele with Archie Brodsky, *Love and Addiction* (New York: NAL/Signet, 1975).

14. James Burkett and Larry Young, "The Behavioral, Anatomical and Pharmacological Parallels Between Social Attachment, Love and Addiction," *Psychopharmacology* 224(1):1–26, 2012, http://www.ncbi.nlm.nih.gov/pubmed/22885871.

15. Lindsay Abrams, "'Sex Addiction' Redefined," *The Atlantic*, October 19, 2012, http://www.theatlantic.com/health/archive/2012/10/sex-addiction-redefined/263873.

16. Pernille Gronkjaer (director), "'Love Addict' Movie Explores Love Addiction, 'Fantasy Universe,'" *Huffington Post,* October 22, 2012, http://www.huffingtonpost.com/2012/10/22/love-addict-movie-explore_n_2002775.html.

17. National Institute on Alcohol Abuse and Alcoholism, "Alcoholism Isn't What It Used to Be," *NIAAA Spectrum*, September 2009, http://www.spectrum.niaaa.nih.gov/media/pdf/NIAAA_Spectrum_Sept_09_tagged.pdf.

18. Shari Roan, "You Can Cut Back," *Los Angeles Times*, November 13, 2009, http://www.latimes.com/features/health/la-he-alcohol16–2009nov16,0,3127580,full.story.

19. Centers for Disease Control and Prevention, "Smoking Cessation: Nicotine Dependence," in *Smoking & Tobacco Use*, http://www.cdc.gov/tobacco/data_statistics/fact_sheets/cessation/quitting/index.htm.

20. Stanton Peele, "This Is How People Quit Addictions," *Huffington Post*, September 13, 2011, http://www.huffingtonpost.com/stanton-peele/this-is-how-people-quit-a_b_949826.html.

21. I could fill this book, as I did my *Addiction-Proof Your Child* (Random House/Three Rivers Press, 2007), with examples and data demonstrating parental remission for alcoholics and drug addicts, like the woman who felt her baby kicking, put down her drink, and said, "I'll never touch another drop," and didn't. Here are two more cases: While discussing Mika Brzezinski's best-selling book on her eating disorder, *Obsessed*, fellow MSNBC host Al Sharpton described how he lost over one hundred pounds (and you think you have a tough addiction to quit?): "My youngest daughter said to me, 'Daddy, why are you so fat?'" Meanwhile, I was at a dinner party with parents of young children. I asked the six parents present if any had smoked—all had. All had quit. I looked at one particularly attentive father of two young children, and said, "I bet you and your wife knew you would sooner kill yourself than not quit"—his wife nodded vigorously.

22. Stanton Peele, "The 7 Hardest Addictions to Quit—Love Is the Worst," *Psychology Today Blogs*, December 15, 2008, http://www.psychologytoday.com/blog/addiction-in-society/200812/the-7-hardest-addictions-quit-love-is-the-worst.

23. Lizzie Crocker, "Mika Brzezinski on 'Obsession,' Her New Book About Food Addiction," *Women in the World*, May 9, 2013, http://www.thedailybeast.com/witw/articles/2013/05/09/mika-brzezinski-on-obsession-her-new-book-about-food-addiction.html.

24. Keith S. Ditman, George G. Crawford, Edward W. Forby et al., "A Controlled Experiment on the Use of Court Probation for Drunk Arrests," *American Journal of Psychiatry* 124:160–163, 1967.

25. Jeffrey Brandsma, Maxie Maultsby, and Richard J. Walsh, *Outpatient Treatment of Alcoholism* (Baltimore: University Park Press, 1980).

26. William R. Miller, Verner S. Westerberg, Richard J. Harris, and J. Scott Tonigan, "What Predicts Relapse? Prospective Testing of Antecedent Models," *Addiction* 91(Supplement):155–171, 1996, http://www.ncbi.nlm.nih.gov/pubmed/8997790.

27. Think New York City—and its population of immigrants—where Prohibition was largely ignored. Mark Lerner, *Dry Manhattan: Prohibition in New York City* (Cambridge, MA: Harvard University Press, 2008).

28. John Kobler, *Ardent Spirits: The Rise and Fall of Prohibition* (New York: Putnam, 1973).

29. Stanton Peele, "Why Medicine for Addiction Will Make Our Problems Worse," *Huffington Post,* July 20, 2011, http://www.huffingtonpost.com/stanton-peele/addiction-medicine-research_b_896744.html.

30. These points were made in the exhibit "American Spirits: The Rise and Fall of Prohibition," at the National Constitution Center in Philadelphia, based on Daniel Okrent's *Last Call*, which also inspired Ken Burns and Lynn Novick's 2011 PBS documentary, *Prohibition*. The exhibit examines "the patchwork of strange liquor laws that began after the repeal of Prohibition and persist to this day. In Oklahoma, no one under 21, not even a baby in its mother's arms, can be in a liquor store; in Indiana, convenience stores can sell beer only at room temperature." Edward Rothstein, "A Look at Prohibition, Hardly Dry," *New York Times*, October 18, 2012, http://www.nytimes.com/2012/10/19/arts/design/american-spirits-at-the-national-constitution-center.html.

31. Stanton Peele, "Alcohol: The Good Side," *Los Angeles Times*, July 21, 2010, http://articles.latimes.com/2010/jul/21/opinion/la-oe-peele-alcohol-20100721.

32. Carl Hart, *High Price: A Neuroscientist's Journey of Self-Discovery That Challenges Everything You Know About Drugs and Society* (New York: HarperCollins, 2013).

33. Douglas Quenqua, "Rethinking Addiction's Roots, and Its Treatment," *New York Times*, July 10, 2011, http://www.nytimes.com/2011/07/11/health/11addictions.html.

34. Stanton Peele, "Addiction in Society: Blinded by Biochemistry," *Psychology Today*, September 1, 2010 http://www.psychologytoday.com/articles/201010/addiction-in-society-blinded-biochemistry.

35. Stanton Peele, "Reductionism in the Psychology of the Eighties: Can Biochemistry Eliminate Addiction, Mental Illness, and Pain?" *American Psychologist* 36:807–818, 1981, http://www.peele.net/lib/reduct.php.

36. Stanton Peele, "You've Got Your Nerves in My Depression," Reason.com, April 30, 2013. Review of Edward Shorter, *How Everyone Became Depressed* (New York: Oxford, 2013), http://reason.com/archives/2013/04/30/youve-got-your-nerves-in-my-depression.

37. Stanton Peele, "The Search for Mental Illness in the Brain, Part I: The Disappointment of the Human Genome Project," *Huffington Post,* May 17, 2013, http://www.huffingtonpost.com/stanton-peele/obama-brain-initiative_b_3286288.html.

38. Abigail Zuger, "A General in the Drug War," *New York Times*, June 13, 2011, http://www.nytimes.com/2011/06/14/science/14volkow.html.

39. Howard Markel, "The D.S.M. Gets Addiction Right," *New York Times*, June 5, 2012, http://www.nytimes.com/2012/06/06/opinion/the-dsm-gets-addiction-right.html.

40. Ian Urbina, "Addiction Diagnoses May Rise Under Guideline Changes," *New York Times*, May 11, 2012, http://www.nytimes.com/2012/05/12/us/dsm-revisions-may-sharply-increase-addiction-diagnoses.html.

41. Maia Szalavitz, "Naomi Wolf's *Vagina* Aside, What Neuroscience Really Says About Female Desire," *Time*, September 18, 2012, http://healthland.time.com/2012/09/18/what-neuroscience-really-says-about-the-vagina-and-female-desire/#ixzz29NoCjxPa.

42. Sam Anderson, "Angry Birds, Farmville and Other Hyperaddictive 'Stupid Games,'" *New York Times Magazine*, April 4, 2012, www.nytimes.com/2012/04/08/magazine/angry-birds-farmville-and-other-hyperaddictive-stupid-games.html.

43. Claire Bates, "Why Only Some People Become Addicted to Drugs: Scans of Cocaine Users Reveal Brain Shape Could Be to Blame," *Mail Online*, January 18, 2013, http://www.dailymail.co.uk/health/article-2264596/Why-people-addicted-drugs-Scans-cocaine-users-reveal-shape-brain-blame.html.

44. Fulton Timm Crews and Charlotte Ann Boettiger, "Impulsivity, Frontal Lobes and Risk for Addiction," *Pharmacology, Biochemistry, and Behavior* 93(3): 237–247, 2009.

45. Joseph LeDoux, *Synaptic Self: How Our Brains Become Who We Are* (New York: Penguin, 2003).

46. Maia Szalavitz, "Siblings Brain Study Sheds Light on Roots of Addiction," *Time*, February 3, 2012, http://healthland.time.com/2012/02/03/siblings-brain-study-sheds-light-on-the-roots-of-addiction.

47. Marnia Robinson and Gary Wilson, "Guys Who Gave Up Porn: On Sex and Romance," *Psychology Today Blogs*, February 1, 2012, http://www.psychologytoday.com/blog/cupids-poisoned-arrow/201202/guys-who-gave-porn-sex-and-romance.

48. Rachael Rettner, "'Sex Addiction' Still Not an Official Disorder," *Livescience*, December 6, 2012, http://www.livescience.com/25306-sex-addiction-disorder.html.

49. Maia Szalavitz, "My Name Is John and I Am a Sex Addict (Or Maybe Not)," *Time*, July 23, 2013, http://healthland.time.com/2013/07/23/my-name-is-john-and-i-am-a-sex-addict-or-maybe-not.

50. Marnia Robinson and Gary Wilson, "Was the Cowardly Lion Just Masturbating Too Much?" *Psychology Today Blogs*, January. 11, 2010, http://www.psychologytoday.com/blog/cupids-poisoned-arrow/201001/was-the-cowardly-lion-just-masturbating-too-much.

51. Robinson and Wilson, "Guys Who Gave Up Porn: On Sex and Romance."

52. Alan Leshner, "Addiction Is a Brain Disease, and It Matters," *Science*, October 3, 278(5335):45–47, 1997.

53. http://vimeo.com/43606271

54. Marc Lewis, "How I Quit. . . . At Least, How I Think I Quit," http://www.memoirsofanaddictedbrain.com/connect/how-i-quit-at-least-how-i-think-i-quit.

55. Maia Szalavitz, "Why the Myth of the Meth-Damaged Brain May Hinder Recovery," *Time*, November 21, 2011, http://healthland.time.com/2011/11/21/why-the-myth-of-the-meth-damaged-brain-may-hinder-recovery.

56. Vincent J. Felitti, "The Origins of Addiction: Evidence from the Adverse Childhood Experiences Study." English version of the article published in Germany as "Ursprünge des Suchtverhaltens—Evidenzen aus einer Studie zu belastenden Kindheitserfahrungen," *Praxis der Kinderpsychologie und Kinderpsychiatrie* 52:547–559, 2003, http://www.acestudy.org/files/OriginsofAddiction.pdf.

57. Norman Doidge, *The Brain That Changes Itself: Stories of Personal Triumph from the Frontiers of Brain Science* (New York: Viking Books, 2007).

58. Stanton Peele, "Dr. Drew, Mindy McCready, and Me," *Psychology Today Blogs*, March 15, 2013, http://www.psychologytoday.com/blog/addiction-in-society/201303/dr-drew-mindy-mccready-and-me.

59. This might be called "free will." But, of course, today the idea that you direct your behavior and control yourself requires a neurological explanation. This has been provided by the iconoclastic but unimpeachable neurological psychologist, Elkhonon Goldberg, who proposes the brain's frontal lobes as the executor of your free will. But *Recover!* is *not* a treatise in philosophy and neuroscience.

60. Andrew Newburg and Mark Robert Waldman, *How God Changes Your Brain: Breakthrough Findings from a Leading Neuroscientist* (New York: Random House, Ballantine, 2010).

61. Kelly McGonigal, *Maximum Willpower: How to Master the New Science of Self-Control* (New York: Macmillan, 2012).

62. Health-care reform—which is absolutely necessary—coupled with parity legislation dictating that mental and addictive problems receive the same coverage as traditional illnesses will inevitably expand the rehab business. And, in the interests of disclosure, as the developer of a treatment program, I have received insurance payments and may well benefit from these further developments.

63. Thomas Rodgers, "Why Do College Students Love Getting Wasted?" *Salon.com*, August 28, 2011, http://www.salon.com/2011/08/28/college_drinking_interview.

64. http://www.hazelden.org/web/public/plymouth_mn_substance_abuse_treatment_center_youth.page

65. "Angelina Jolie: Humanitarian," *Time*, May 14, 2013, http://entertainment.time.com/2013/05/14/angelina-jolie-humanitarian.

66. "Angelina Jolie Biography," *Scribe Town*, December 30, 2011, http://www.scribe-town.com/angelina-jolie-biography.

67. Chris Laxamana, "#050: Dr. Adi Jaffe and Dr. Marc Kern," *DrDrew*, May 17, 2013. In this remarkable podcast, Dr. Drew interviews two leading practitioners of harm reduction, including the idea that many former addicts can use substances

safely again. Dr. Drew repeatedly asserts that he is "a scientist," while trying to explain away the reality of the information provided by Drs. Jaffe and Kern, including their own life experiences. http://drdrew.com/050-dr-adi-jaffe-and-dr-marc-kern.

68. NIAAA, "Alcoholism Isn't What It Used to Be."

69. Deborah A. Dawson, Bridget F. Grant, Frederick S. Stinson, et al., "Recovery from DSM-IV Alcohol Dependence, United States, 2001–2002," *Addiction* 100:281–292, 2005.

70. Bridget F. Grant and Deborah A. Dawson, "Introduction to the National Epidemiologic Survey on Alcohol and Related Conditions," *National Institute of Alcohol Abuse and Alcoholism Publications*, http://pubs.niaaa.nih.gov/publications/arh29-2/74-78.htm.

71. Effectiveness Bank Bulletin, "Findings," October 30, 2013, http://findings.org.uk/docs/bulletins/Bull_30_10_13.php. This bulletin incorporated the following three studies: Catalina Lopez-Quintero, Deborah S. Hasin, José Pérez de los Cobos, et al. "Probability and Predictors of Remission from Life-Time Nicotine, Alcohol, Cannabis or Cocaine Dependence: Results from the National Epidemiologic Survey on Alcohol and Related Conditions," *Addiction* 106(3):657–669, 2011; Gene Heyman, "Quitting Drugs: Quantitative and Qualitative Features," *Annual Review of Clinical Psychology* 9:29–59, 2013; William L. White, *Recovery/Remission from Substance Use Disorders: An Analysis of Reported Outcomes in 415 Scientific Reports, 1868–2011* (Great Lakes Addiction Technology Transfer Center, Philadelphia Department of Behavioral Health and Intellectual Disability Services, and Northeast Addiction Technology Transfer Center, 2012).

72. Substance Abuse and Mental Health Services Administration, "Substance Dependence or Abuse in the Past Year, by Detailed Age Category: Percentages, 2011," *National Survey on Drug Use and Health*, Table 5.3B, http://www.samhsa.gov/data/NSDUH/2011SummNatFindDetTables/NSDUH-DetTabsPDFWHTML2011/2k11DetailedTabs/Web/HTML/NSDUH-DetTabsSect5peTabs1to56-2011.htm#Tab5.3B.

73. Stanton Peele, "Addiction: The Analgesic Experience," *Human Nature*, September, 1978, http://www.peele.net/lib/analgesic.php.

74. Lee M. Robins et al., "Drug Use by U.S. Army Enlisted Men in Vietnam: A Follow-Up on Their Return Home," *American Journal of Epidemiology* 99:235–249, 1974.

75. Harold Mulford, one of the great researchers and thinkers in the alcoholism/addiction field, said it first: "Contrary to the traditional clinical view of the alcoholism disease process, progress in the alcoholic process is neither inevitable nor irreversible. Eventually, the balance of natural forces shifts to decelerate progress in the alcoholic process and to accelerate the rehabilitation process."

"Rethinking the Alcohol Problem: A Natural Processes Model," *Journal of Drug Issues* 14:38, 1984.

76. William R. Miller, Paula L. Wilbourne, and Jennifer E. Hettema, "What Works? A Summary of Alcohol Treatment Outcome Research," in Reid K. Hester and William R. Miller, eds., *Handbook of Alcoholism Treatment Approaches: Effective Alternatives*, 3rd ed. (Boston: Allyn & Bacon, 2003), pp. 13–63.

77. William R. Miller, Allen Zweben, and Bruce Johnson, "Evidence-Based Treatment," *Journal of Substance Abuse Treatment* 29:267–276, 2005, http://www.ncbi.nlm.nih.gov/pubmed/16311179.

78. Linda Brown et al., "Participant Perspectives on Mindfulness Meditation Training for Anxiety in Schizophrenia," *American Journal of Psychiatric Rehabilitation* 13(3):224–242, 2010, http://www.tandfonline.com/doi/abs/10.1080/15487768.2010.501302.

79. Paula DeSanto, *Effective Addiction Treatment: The Minnesota Alternative* (Minnesota: Minnesota Alternatives, 2012), http://mnalternatives.com/products.

80. Sarah Bowen et al., "Mindfulness-Based Relapse Prevention for Substance Use Disorders: A Pilot Efficacy Trial," *Substance Abuse* 30(4):295–305, 2009. This work is from Alan Marlatt's group at the University of Washington. This book is dedicated to Alan's memory.

Chapter 3

1. The HAMS (Harm Reduction for Alcohol) Network, under Kenneth Anderson, has developed valuable materials for assessing and going through withdrawal. HAMS regards the most medically risky withdrawal as occurring with alcohol and benzodiazapines (tranquilizers). "What Is Alcohol Withdrawal?" http://hamsnetwork.org/withdrawal. In the case of alcohol, major withdrawal (delirium tremens, which is marked by hallucinations) is most clearly life threatening, although the mid-level withdrawal Alex underwent is likewise medically challenging. "Less than 50% of alcohol-dependent persons develop any significant withdrawal symptoms that require pharmacologic treatment upon cessation of alcohol intake. The lifetime risk for developing delirium tremens (DTs) among chronic alcoholics is estimated at 5–10%. Only 5% of patients with ethanol withdrawal progress to delirium tremens." "Delirium Tremens," Medscape, http://emedicine.medscape.com/article/166032-overview#a0156. HAMS provides guidance on your likelihood of undergoing withdrawal. "The Odds of Going Through Alcohol Withdrawal," http://hamsnetwork.org/odds. Whatever these risks, people undergo medically unsupervised alcohol withdrawal all the time. For people doing so, HAMS recommends tapering (drinking lesser amounts to suppress withdrawal—in medical settings, doctors nearly always administer benzodiazapines to accomplish the same purpose). "How To Taper Off Alcohol," http://hamsnetwork.org/taper. And, of

course, people need a backup plan should they begin to show serious withdrawal symptoms.

2. Jane Gross, "Plan to Become an Ex-Smoker for Good," *New York Times*, November 12, 2012, http://well.blogs.nytimes.com/2012/11/12/plan-to-become-an-ex-smoker-for-good.

3. Alan Marlatt and his colleagues have amply demonstrated this. See Mary E. Larimer, Rebekka S. Palmer, and G. Alan Marlatt, "Relapse Prevention: An Overview of Marlatt's Cognitive-Behavioral Model," *Alcohol Research and Health* 23(2):151–60, 1999, http://www.ncbi.nlm.nih.gov/pubmed/10890810.

4. Substance Abuse and Mental Health Services Administration, "News Release: A Working Definition of 'Recovery' from Mental Disorders and Substance Use Disorders," December 22, 2011, http://www.samhsa.gov/newsroom/advisories/1112223420.aspx.

5. Substance Abuse and Mental Health Services Administration, "Recovery Defined—A Unified Working Definition and Set of Principles," May 20, 2011, http://blog.samhsa.gov/2011/05/20/recovery-defined-a-unified-working-definition-and-set-of-principles.

6. Alex Copello, Jim Orford, Ray Hodgson, and Gillian Tober, *Social Behaviour and Network Therapy for Alcohol Problems* (London: Routledge, 2009). In a trial, SBNT and motivational enhancement therapy were compared—the treatments had equal efficacy as measured by improved mental health and quality of life, decreased alcohol use and dependence, and fewer secondary problems. http://bjp.rcpsych.org/content/197/3/251.2.full.

7. Stanton Peele, "The 7 Hardest Addictions to Quit: Love Is the Worst!," *Psychology Today Blogs*, December 15, 2008. http://www.psychologytoday.com/blog/addiction-in-society/200812/the-7-hardest-addictions-quit-love-is-the-worst.

8. Rachel Yoder, "Strung Out on Love and Checked In for Treatment," *New York Times*, June 11, 2006, www.nytimes.com/2006/06/11/fashion/sundaystyles/11love.html.

9. Stanton Peele, *The Meaning of Addiction* (Lexington, MA: Lexington Books, 1985; San Francisco: Jossey-Bass, 1998), http://www.peele.net/lib/moa1.php.

10. Pamela Druckerman, *Bringing Up Bébé* (New York, Penguin, 2012). See review by Susannah Meadows, "Raising the Perfect Child, with Time for Smoke Breaks," *New York Times*, February 7, 2012, http://www.nytimes.com/2012/02/08/books/bringing-up-bebe-a-french-influenced-guide-by-pamela-druckerman.html.

11. Roy F. Baumeister and John Tierney, *Willpower: Rediscovering the Greatest Human Strength* (New York: Penguin Books, 2012).

12. Sandra Aamodt and Sam Wang, "Building Self-Control, the American Way," *New York Times*, February 17, 2012, www.nytimes.com/2012/02/19/opinion/sunday/building-self-control-the-american-way.html.

13. Kate Taylor, "Council Speaker Recounts Her Struggles with Bulimia and Alcoholism," *New York Times*, May 14, 2013, http://www.nytimes.com/2013/05/14/nyregion/council-speaker-opens-up-about-her-struggles-against-bulimia-and-alcoholism.html.

14. Andrew Goldman, "Billy Joel on Not Working and Not Giving Up Drinking," *New York Times Magazine*, May 26, 2013, www.nytimes.com/2013/05/26/magazine/billy-joel-on-not-working-and-not-giving-up-drinking.html.

15. Chris Laxamana, "#050: Dr. Adi Jaffe and Dr. Marc Kern," *DrDrew*, May 17, 2013. In this remarkable podcast, Dr. Drew interviews two leading practitioners of harm reduction, including the idea that many former addicts can use substances safely again. Dr. Drew repeatedly asserts that he is "a scientist," while trying to explain away the reality of the information provided by Drs. Jaffe and Kern, including their own life experiences. http://drdrew.com/050-dr-adi-jaffe-and-dr-marc-kern.

16. Kenneth Anderson, "First Do No Harm," *The Fix*, March 27, 2013, http://thefix.com/content/harm-reduction-alcohol-HMAS-moderation-drinking8008.

17. Kenneth Anderson, "Alcohol Harm Reduction Compared to Harm Reduction for Other Drugs," Presented at the Ninth National Harm Reduction Conference, Portland, OR, November 16, 2012, http://hamsnetwork.org/9th-conference/compared.pdf.

18. Megan McLemore, "A Step Backward for AIDS Prevention," *Huffington Post*, August 28, 2012, http://www.huffingtonpost.com/megan-mclemore/a-step-backward-for-aids-prevention_b_1831504.html.

19. Harm reduction therapy for even intense drug users has been spearheaded by Patt Denning, Jeannie Little, and Adina Glickman, *Over the Influence: The Harm Reduction Guide for Managing Drugs and Alcohol* (New York: Guilford, 2004).

20. Nick Heather and Ian Robertson, *Controlled Drinking* (New York: Routledge, 1984).

Chapter 4

1. Ellen J. Langer, *Mindfulness* (Cambridge, MA: Perseus, 1989).

2. U.C.L.A. Mindful Awareness Center, http://marc.ucla.edu/body.cfm?id=19; University of Massachusetts Medical School Center for Mindfulness, http://w3.umassmed.edu/MBSR/public/searchmember.aspx.

3. National Cancer Institute, *Smoking and Tobacco Control Monograph Series #15: Those Who Continue to Smoke* (Washington, DC: National Institutes of Health, 2003), http://cancercontrol.cancer.gov/brp/tcrb/monographs/15/index.html.

4. Sarah Bowen, Neha Chawla, and G. Alan Marlatt, *Mindfulness-Based Relapse Prevention for Addictive Behaviors: A Clinician's Guide* (New York: Guilford, 2011).

5. Pavel Somov, *Eating the Moment: 141 Mindful Practices to Overcome Overeating One Meal at a Time* (Oakland, CA: New Harbinger, 2008).

6. Abby Ellin, "Fat and Thin Find Common Ground," *New York Times*, October 10, 2013 http://www.well.blogs.nytimes.com/2013/10/10/can-the-fat-and-thin-just-get-along.

7. Stanton Peele, "Addiction in Society: Blinded by Biochemistry," *Psychology Today*, September 1, 2010 http://www.psychologytoday.com/articles/201010/addiction-in-society-blinded-biochemistry.

8. Sarah Bowen et al., "Mindfulness-Based Relapse Prevention for Substance Use Disorders: A Pilot Efficacy Trial," *Substance Abuse* 30:205–305, 2009.

Chapter 5

1. Maia Szalavitz, "Being Ashamed of Drinking Prompts Relapse, Not Recovery," *Time*, February 7, 2013, http://healthland.time.com/2013/02/07/being-ashamed-of-drinking-prompts-relapse-not-recovery.

2. William L. White and William R. Miller, "The Use of Confrontation in Addiction Treatment: History, Science and Time for Change," *Counselor* 8(4): 12–30, 2007.

3. Alcoholics Anonymous World Organization, *Step One: "We admitted we were powerless over alcohol."* New York: AA World Services, www.aa.org/twelveandtwelve/en_pdfs/en_step1.pdf.

4. National Center for Mental Health Checkups, Columbia University, *Teens and Eating Disorders* (New York: Columbia University, 2013), http://www.teenscreen.org/resources/eating-disorders.

5. Ken Anderson, "First Do No Harm," *The Fix*, March 27, 2013, http://thefix.com/content/harm-reduction-alcohol-HMAS-moderation-drinking8008.

6. James Robert Milam and Katherine Ketchum, *Under the Influence* (New York: Bantam, 1981).

7. Bob Egelko, "Appeals Court Says Requirement to Attend AA Unconstitutional," *San Francisco Chronicle*, September 7, 2007, http://www.sfgate.com/bayarea/article/Appeals-court-says-requirement-to-attend-AA-2542005.php#ixzz2UKKobB00.

8. Helen Y. Yang, Andrew S. Fox, Alexander J. Shackman et al., "Compassion Training Alters Altruism and Neural Responses to Suffering," *Psychological Science*, May 21, 2013, http://pss.sagepub.com/content/early/2013/05/20/0956797612469537.abstract.

9. Kelly McGonigal, *The Willpower Instinct: How Self-Control Works, Why It Matters, and What You Can Do to Get More of It* (New York: Penguin, 2012).

10. Alex Witchel, "How Jeannette Walls Spins Good Stories Out of Bad Memories," *New York Times*, May 24, 2013, www.nytimes.com/2013/05/26/magazine/how-jeannette-walls-spins-good-stories-out-of-bad-memories.html.

Chapter 6

1. Roy F. Baumeister and John Tierney, *Willpower: Rediscovering the Greatest Human Strength* (New York: Penguin Books, 2012). The book is filled with complicated brain, neurochemical, and evolutionary psychology analyses—indeed, the book stands as an illustration of how speculative and unhelpful such notions are when applied to a common-sense idea.

2. James O. Prochaska and Carlo DiClemente, *The Transtheoretical Approach: Towards a Systematic Eclectic Framework* (Homewood, IL: Dow Jones Irwin, 1984).

Chapter 7

1. G. Alan Marlatt and Dennis M. Donovan, *Relapse Prevention, Second Edition: Maintenance Strategies in the Treatment of Addictive Behaviors* (New York: Guilford, 2005).

2. Roy F. Baumeister and John Tierney, *Willpower: Rediscovering the Greatest Human Strength* (New York: Penguin Books, 2012).

3. John Tierney, "Why You Won't Be the Person You Expect to Be," *New York Times*, January 3, 2013, www.nytimes.com/2013/01/04/science/study-in-science-shows-end-of-history-illusion.html.

4. Alex Copello, Jim Orford, Ray Hodgson et al., "Social Behaviour and Network Therapy: Basic Principles and Early Experience," *Addictive Behaviors* 27(3):345–366, 2002.

5. In the interest of a spouse or loved one's not only getting out of the way, but being a support for overcoming addiction, PERFECT opposes current 12-step thinking. AA and its derivatives have complex differences in how they view spouses of alcoholics. Alanon is a group for spouses (nearly always meaning wives) of alcoholics that is famous for telling members it's the alcoholic's problem and the wife's only chance to survive is by understanding that her husband is diseased. "You can't control your alcoholic spouse" is the Alanon mantra. "Don't try." By Alanon's lights, William should leave Sabrina to her own devices (meaning she had better go to AA) and look out for himself. More recently, however, has come the idea of codependence (distantly related to the idea of love addiction I have developed). Codependents—again, *usually* women—have a disease just like the alcoholic or drug addict—only the object of their disease is the addicted person. In codependence terms, Sabrina and William have equivalent, supporting diseases against which each of them must struggle by working the 12 steps!

6. The indexes for both *Tools* and *Truth* list a number of places where the community reinforcement approach (CRA)—including reciprocity marital counseling—is discussed.

7. Pavel Somov, *Present Perfect: A Mindfulness Approach to Letting Go of Perfectionism and the Need for Control* (Oakland, CA: New Harbinger, 2010).

8. Susan Sontag, *Regarding the Pain of Others* (New York: Picador, 2003).

9. Warren St. John, "Sorrow So Sweet," *New York Times*, August 24, 2002, www.nytimes.com/2002/08/24/arts/sorrow-so-sweet-a-guilty-pleasure-in-another-s-woe.html.

10. William L. White and William R. Miller, "The Use of Confrontation in Addiction Treatment: History, Science and Time for Change," *Counselor* 8(4):12–30, 2007.

11. Maia Szalavitz, *Help at Any Cost: How the Troubled-Teen Industry Cons Parents and Hurts Kids* (New York: Riverhead, 2006).

12. Robert J. Meyers and Brenda L. Wolfe, *Get Your Loved One Sober: Alternatives to Nagging, Pleading, and Threatening* (Center City, MN: Hazelden, 2004).

13. Maia Szalavitz, "Is Dr. Drew Too Dangerous for Prime Time?" *The Fix*, February 25, 2012, http://www.salon.com/2013/02/25/is_dr_drew_too_dangerous_for_prime_time.

14. Stanton Peele and Alan Cudmore, "Intervene This," *Huffington Post*, January 23, 2012, http://www.huffingtonpost.com/stanton-peele/addiction-intervention_b_1220753.html.

15. William R. Miller, Robert J. Meyers, and J. Scott Tonigan, "Engaging the Unmotivated in Treatment for Alcohol Problems: A Comparison of Three Strategies for Intervention Through Family Members," *Journal of Consulting and Clinical Psychology* 67: 688–97, 1999.

16. William R. Miller and Stephen Rollnick, *Motivational Interviewing, Third Edition: Helping People Change* (New York: Guilford Press, 2013).

Chapter 8

1. Roy F. Baumeister and John Tierney, *Willpower: Rediscovering the Greatest Human Strength* (New York: Penguin Books, 2012).

2. The best book about assessing potential addiction treatment facilities and therapists is Anne M. Fletcher, *Inside Rehab: The Surprising Truth About Addiction Treatment—And How to Get Help That Works* (New York: Viking, 2013).

3. G. Alan Marlatt, ed., *Harm Reduction: Pragmatic Strategies for Managing High-Risk Behaviors*, 2nd ed. (New York: Guilford, 1998).

4. Stanton Peele and Bruce K. Alexander, "Theories of Addiction," in Stanton Peele, *The Meaning of Addiction*, 2nd ed. (San Francisco: Jossey-Bass, 1998), pp. 47–72; http://lifeprocessprogram.com/the-meaning-of-addiction-3-theories-of-addiction.

5. Sarah Bowen, Neha Chawla, and G. Alan Marlatt, *Mindfulness-Based Relapse Prevention for Addictive Behaviors: A Clinician's Guide* (New York: Guilford, 2011).

6. There are now many books and programs on this topic. See Thich Nht Hanh and Lilian Cheung, *Savor: Mindful Eating, Mindful Life* (New York: Harper, 2011).

Chapter 9

1. Maia Szalavitz, "Being Ashamed of Drinking Prompts Relapse, Not Recovery," *Time*, February 7, 2013, http://healthland.time.com/2013/02/07/being-ashamed-of-drinking-prompts-relapse-not-recovery.

2. nonajordan.com

Index

About the Authors

Stanton Peele has been a cutting-edge figure in the addiction field for four decades since the publication of *Love and Addiction* in 1975. He has been a pioneer in noting addiction across substances and activities, in creating harm reduction therapy, and in the nondisease understanding of addiction, as well as in formulating practical, life-management approaches to treatment and self-help. Stanton has written 12 books (including *The Meaning of Addiction*, *Diseasing of America*, *The Truth About Addiction and Recovery*, *7 Tools to Beat Addiction*, and *Addiction-Proof Your Child*) and 250 professional articles, won numerous awards (including from the Rutgers Center of Alcohol Studies and the Drug Policy Alliance), and created the Life Process Program for addiction treatment, which continues to be utilized worldwide. Stanton also lectures on addiction around the world. He has blogged as an addiction expert for *The Fix*, *Psychology Today*, *Reason*, *Substance.com*, and *The Huffington Post*. He was named the best addiction blogger by All Treatment and one of the ten most influential figures in the addiction field by *The Fix*.

Ilse Thompson is a writer and editor living in Portland, Oregon. She is pursuing her Master of Divinity in Buddhism at Maitripa College.

Made in the USA
Las Vegas, NV
05 March 2022

45045008R00185